1

Integrating Modern Medicine with Yoga and Ayurveda for Better Patient Care

By Dr Rajeev Gupta

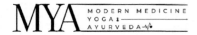

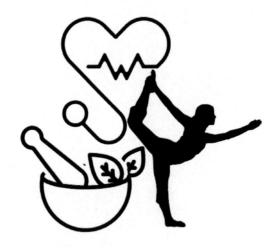

© Dr Rajeev Gupta

Acknowledgments

I would like to express my heartfelt gratitude to all those who contributed to the creation of this book.

First, I am deeply grateful to my teachers in the fields of modern medicine, yoga, and Ayurveda, who have generously shared their knowledge and wisdom with me. You have shaped my understanding of health and wellbeing and instilled in me a deep respect for these disciplines. I am especially thankful to Dr B D Gupta for instilling enthusiasm for medicine that is still going after 30 years.

I am grateful to my wife for supporting me all through my journey and compassionate to me for not giving her time that she deserved while I was dedicating time to research the facts and write the book. I am also grateful to my sister who has been a source of inspiration and support all my life.

I am also grateful to my children, family and friends, your unwavering support and encouragement have meant the world to me. You have been my rock throughout this journey.

I am also grateful to my colleagues, your intellectual camaraderie and collaborative spirit have been invaluable. Your insights, questions, and shared experiences have enriched my perspective and informed my writing. I am also thankful to my patients and students, thank you for your trust and for allowing me to be part of your health journey. Your stories, struggles, and successes have been a constant source of inspiration.

I am eternally grateful to my readers, thank you for your interest in this topic and for supporting me in this mission of integrating modern medicine with other healthcare disciplines for a better patient care. It's a long journey, however keeping you in mind I have put all the efforts I admire your commitment to new health horizon. It is for you that this book was written. I am grateful to my team who have worked hard to bring this book into a good shape.

I am eternally grateful to Swami Ramdev ji who has transformed the life of millions of people and has brought the yoga into everyday practice for population at large. He has been instrumental in my yoga journey and has further inspired me giving the responsibility to be the head of the medical advisory board of the PYPT UK

Special thanks and acknowledgements to Shri Balkrishan ji and Dr Anurag Varnsley for helping to shape this book effectively.

Finally heartfelt thanks to Sunita Poddar ji and PYPT UK for the help in bringing this book live at a short notice.

Dedicated to my mother who was the source of my inspiration and she always inspired me to think differently and go beyond the norms.

Why I wrore this book about integrating Modern Medicine, Yoga and Ayurveda

Having read a lot about and explored the principles of modern medicine, yoga, and Ayurveda, I have come to realise that there is a difference in approach of these systems and therefore we have not been able to take the advantage of combining the ancient medicine what worked well for centuries, and modern medicine which is new evidence-based and authentic but expensive health care technology.

If however we can try to understand the approach of the system and bring a synergy of these practices with their unique perspectives and methodologies, we can brings something different to the healthcare table.

Modern medicine excels at diagnosing and treating acute conditions and managing chronic diseases. It offers powerful tools for rapid symptom relief and lifesaving interventions. Its strength lies in its scientific rigor, its ability to standardize treatments, and its focus on disease pathology.

On the other hand, yoga offers a preventive approach to health, with physical, mental, and spiritual benefits. The body posture and gentle stretching movements (asanas) bring improvement of bone   and joint health, but altho contru#ibutes to overall physical health. The Breathing Exercises (Pranayams) help improving the air flow, the deep diapgraphmatic breathing improve the lung functions and overall oxygenation of tissues to improve vitality. The medictation techniques can calm the mind, and instil a sense of inner peace and balance. Its emphasis on mindfulness and self-care empowers individuals to play an active role in their health and is second to none for stress management which is a big contrinuting factor to the modern diseases.

Ayurveda, with its holistic and individual-centric view of health, offers personalised wellness strategies. Its focus on balancing the mind, body, and spirit, and its preventive approach, aligns well with contemporary understanding of wellness and chronic disease management. The jhealthy foods with alteration of diet pattern and life style helps and contribute further to the disease management in modern medicine. Additional benefits of the plant derived products have significant contribution to the chronic disease management.

Together, these systems can offer a multi-dimensional approach to health, providing comprehensive care that improves patient outcomes and satisfaction. By acknowledging and integrating the strengths of each system, we can move towards a model of health that is person-centred, holistic, and empowering.

The goal of this integrated approach is not to replace one system with another but to find the most effective combination for each individual. It's about respecting the uniqueness of each person, their health condition, and their personal beliefs and preferences.

The beauty of this integration lies in its flexibility and adaptability. There is a choice and it can be tailored to meet the unique needs and preferences of each individual. This personalised approach not only improves health outcomes but also enhances the individual's engagement and satisfaction with their healthcare.

Integrating modern medicine with yoga and Ayurveda doesn't mean disregarding the science that underpins modern healthcare. Instead, it invites us to expand our understanding of health, to include not just the physical but also the mental, emotional, and spiritual dimensions.

As we continue on this journey, we'll explore this integrated approach further, delving into practical guidelines, real-life case studies, and scientific evidence. The goal is to provide a comprehensive understanding of how these systems can work together to promote optimal health and wellness.

It's important to note that while this integrated approach offers many benefits, it's not a magic bullet. Just like any other healthcare approach, it requires commitment, consistency, and patience. Moreover, it should be guided by qualified healthcare professionals to ensure safety and effectiveness.

The path towards optimal health is a personal journey, one that is unique to each of us. By combining the best of modern medicine, yoga, and Ayurveda, we can empower ourselves to navigate this journey with wisdom, balance, and resilience. Together, these practices can light the way towards a more holistic, integrative understanding of health and wellbeing.

Remember, health is a journey, not a destination. May this book be a helpful guide on your journey to optimal health and wellness. Your path is unique, and your potential is boundless. Embrace the journey, and cherish each step along the way.

Dr Rajeev Gupta, MBBS, MD, MRCP (UK), FRCPCH (UK), MBA, DECC, AEQi

Consultant Paediatrician,
Chairman Central Specialist Committee, Royal College of Paediatrics and Child Health,
Ex-Chairman of the Regional Council of British medical Association,
Ex-Chairman Regional Consultants Committee, BMA
Director, International Organisation of Integrated Health Practitioners
Head of Medical Advisory Board, Patanjali Yog Peeth Trust UK

Preface

In the aftermath of writing this book, I am left with a deep sense of gratitude and hope. Gratitude for the wisdom of the ages and the discoveries of modern science that have paved the way for the integrative approach to healthcare we explored. Hope for the future, where the integration of modern medicine, yoga, and Ayurveda might become more commonplace, enabling individuals to live healthier, happier, and more balanced lives.

The dialogue between the old and the new, the East and the West, the physical and the spiritual, is not always an easy one. It is filled with challenges and complexities. However, it is a dialogue that holds immense potential for enriching our understanding of health and improving the ways we care for ourselves and each other.

As we stand at this crossroads of healthcare, we have a unique opportunity to shape its future. By embracing a more holistic, integrative approach, we can foster a healthcare system that truly caters to the whole person. A system that not only treats illness but also promotes health and wellbeing.

Although modern medicine is most accepted worldwide, however there is no cure for all diseases in this or any other discipline including alternative and complementary medicine. I believe that if we can combine the best parts of modern , complementary and alternative medicine, we can provide highest quality of care to the patient. International Organisation of Integrated Health Practitioners is trying to combine conventional modern medicine with yoga, Ayurveda, TaiChi, Qigong, homeopathy, Acupuncture, Acupressure, Hypnotherapy, Chiropractice, Massage therapy, aromatherapy, dance therapy, music therapy, art therapy etc. Since combining all is quite a herculean task, particularly because I want to do it in in an evidence based way, I have decided to take smaller chunks. This book is a piece of combining modern conventional medicine with yoga and Ayurveda.

The book has fundamentals of systems and areas of convergence of the disciplines which were thought dissimilar and far apart, however I have tried to bring them together to have some taste and consider possibility of combining these for a better quality of life, preservation of health and cost-effectiveness.

The book as 3 parts, the first part introduce modern medicine, yoga and Ayurveda with their uniqueness and commonness. Second part takes each body system on its own, and analyse the perspective of modern medicine, yoga and Ayurveda followed by understanding of a combined effect. Part three brings together with practical implications and examples in different diseases, the benefit of synergy, discussion about methodology of integration and with impact with a cost-benefit analysis.

It's a new and different, but I invite you to join me in this endeavour. Let's continue to learn, grow, and evolve. Let's be curious, open-minded, and proactive in our pursuit of health and wellbeing. And most importantly, let's care for ourselves and each other with compassion, respect, and love.

Although I have held various positions in a variety of governmental and non-governmental positions, the views expressed in this book are my own and based on my thinking and experience.

I have had the western medical training, had been practicing as consultant in the United Kingdom over two decades but opted to have a deep dive into yoga and Ayurveda because there is no cure for every disease, and I was looking for alternatives. Patanjali Yog Peeth Trust UK has been the source of inspiration for me and have supported me in the quest. I have read a lot and connected my scientific medical knowledge to the practical aspects of asanas, breathing exercises and meditation.I looked into the potential benefits and scientific reasoning for the benefits in detail. I have been fortunate to have done the yoga teacher training and be with the group of yoga teachers to share and reflect on the experience. Swami Ramdev ji have appointed me to be the Head Medical Advisory Board of PYPT UK and we have done a lot of work explaining health benefits of yoga in a scientific way that is acceptable to the UK population. We are not undermining the value of any health care discipline, we are trying to bring all disciplines together so that the population at large and the patients can have benefit of all 3, modern medicine, yoga and Ayurveda in an evidence-based fashion. Health is not merely absence of disease, and has physical, mental and emotional components which can be more effectively managed by the combination.

Good health is not a destination but a journey, understanding and enjoying the journey allows more profound benefits. I wish you enjoy a better health and help your family and friends to do the same. Cherish this journey and continue to seek out ways to nurture your body, mind, and spirit.

May this book serve as a stepping stone on your path to optimal health and wellness. May it inspire you, empower you, and guide you towards a life of balance, vitality, and peace.

With warm regards,

Dr Rajeev Gupta, MBBS, MD, MRCP (UK), FRCPCH (UK), MBA, DECC, AEQi

Consultant Paediatrician,
Chairman Central Specialist Committee, Royal College of Paediatrics and Child Health,
Ex-Chairman of the Regional Council of British medical Association,
Ex-Chairman Regional Consultants Committee, BMA
Director, International Organisation of Integrated Health Practitioners
Head of Medical Advisory Board, Patanjali Yog Peeth Trust UK

About the Author

Dr Rajeev Gupta is a qualified medical doctor with over 35 years of experience. He has lived in india for almost 3 decades in India and learned the modern medicine as well as Ayurveda, Yoga, Homeopathy and other ancient sciences while doing his graduate and post-graduate medical qualification. He has further dived deep while practising as medical doctor in the United Kingdom for almost 3 decaes and has tried to understand the quality care, research based evidence creation and universality of practices for quality patient care. He has been clinical audit lead for over 10 years and has understood how the clinical care should be refined by understanding the gaps and creating guidelines and revising guidelines.

He has however also observed and experienced about the patient care being fragmented due to specialisation and sub-specialisation of the modern meeicine. The patient at times get forgotten in the journey as doctors get more specialist intheir area.

There is however a bigger gap in the care of chronic diseases due to single system of care i.e. modern or western medicine also called allopathy and for example a patient with chronic pain or fibfomylagia just getting pain killers, and stronger pain killers when visit Gp or specialist to the extent that side effects on kidney or other systems appear.

No one system of medical care has cure for all diseases and it makes sense if we can bring some harmony. Dr Gupta having huge experience of different systems but also huge enthusiasm and passion to bring these together for a better patient care is an example of his uniqueness and dedication. He is a seasoned professional with extensive experience in the field of health and wellness. With a multidisciplinary background that includes modern medicine, yoga, and Ayurveda, he has uniquely equipped to bridge these systems and offer an integrated perspective on health and wellbeing. His writing is informed by a deep knowledge of scientific rigor, a commitment to holistic healthcare, and a passion for helping others improve their health and quality of life.

A lifelong learner, the author believes in the importance of staying up-to-date with the latest research and developments in healthcare. Diving deep into this field with ongoing learning allowed him to continually refine his understanding and approach, ensuring that he provides the most relevant, effective guidance to the readers.

Dr Rajeev Gupta is a name known in field if medicine not just in the Uk but across the globe due to his involvement in Healing Our Earth programme which started during the Covid-19 pandemic. He has been chairman of of the Central Specialist Committee of the Royal College of Paediatrics and Child Health, Chairamn of the Regional Council of the British medical Association, Chairman of the Regional Consultant Committee of the British Medical Assi#ociation, Chairman of the Education Committee of the British Society of Paediatric Gastroenterology, Hepatology and Nutrition , and also the Director of Internatiional Organisation of Intergrated Health Practitioners.

His courage and stamina to go beyond his western medicine career to look deep into the science behind yoga and Ayurveda make him unique. Having understood different disciplines of health care, he has started building the bridges and bringing these together on commonness principles. His commitment to holistic health and integrated medicine extends beyond his professional life. He personally practice the principles he preaches, incorporating yoga and Ayurveda into his lifestyle and combining it with modern medicine for his healthcare needs. This personal experience enriches his professional perspective, allowing him to offer practical, first hand advice.

He is highly talents and received multiple clinical excellence awards from the National Health Service of the United Kingdom, also received multiple other award including outstanding personal achievement award, personal service award, and the Award for Integration at World TaiChi and Qigong Cogress 2022. He also received Health Care Leadership Award by World Book of Awards at the British Parliament recently in 2022. He is deeply honoured to share his insights with you and hope this book serves as a valuable resource on your health journey. He invites you to approach this exploration with an open mind, a curious spirit, and a commitment to your wellbeing.

CONTENTS

Why I wrote this book about integrating Modern Medicine, Yoga and Ayurveda   5

Introduction   13

PART-1

Viewing health from the perspective of Modern Medicine   17

Understanding health from the perspective of Yoga   20

Understanding Ayurveda the ancient art of healing   23

Practical implementation of Integrative approach   27

Practical examples of integrated approach   28

Commonness in principles of Modern Medicine, Yoga and Ayurveda   31

Harmonisation of Modern Medicine, Yoga and Ayurveda   33

Addressing concerns in integrating Modern Medicine, Yoga and Ayurveda   34

Benefits of integration of Modern Medicine, Yoga and Ayurveda   36

The Journey of Integration   38

PART-2

Respiratory system - approach of Modern Medicine, Yoga and Ayurveda   42

Nervous system - approach of Modern Medicine, Yoga and Ayurveda   52

Endocrine system - approach of Modern med Medicine, Yoga and Ayurveda   60

Cardio-vascular system - approach of Modern Medicine, Yoga and Ayurveda   70

Renal and urinary system - approach of Modern Medicine, Yoga and Ayurveda   79

Reproductive system – male - approach of Modern Medicine, Yoga and Ayurveda   86

Reproductive system – female - approach of Modern Medicine, Yoga and Ayurveda   95

Bones and joints - approach of Modern Medicine, Yoga and Ayurveda   103

Mental health problems - approach of Modern Medicine, Yoga and Ayurveda   110

Digestive system - approach of Modern Medicine, Yoga and Ayurveda   119

Haematology - approach of Modern Medicine, Yoga and Ayurveda 125

Immunity and Infections - approach of Modern Medicine, Yoga and Ayurveda 132

Dermatology - approach of Modern Medicine, Yoga and Ayurveda 141

Surgical conditions - approach of Modern Medicine, Yoga and Ayurveda 147

Dental and oral diseases - approach of Modern Medicine, Yoga and Ayurveda 154

PART-3

Synergy of Modern Medicine, Yoga and Ayurveda 161

Practical Examples of Diseases with Synergistic approach for Better patient care 164

Diabetes, Hypertension, Chronic Arthritis, Dementia, Chronic Asthma, COPD, Migraine, Inflammatory Bowel Disease, Irritable Bowel Syndrome, Obesity, Chronic Eczema, Dysmenorrhoea, Chronic Fatigue Syndrome, Systemic Lupus Erythematosus, Multiple Sclerosis, Fibromyalgia, Hypothyroidism, Hyperthyroidism, Anxiety Disorder, Depression, ADHD, Insomnia, Anorexia Nervosa, Allergic conditions, Alzheimer's Disease, Parkinsonism, Sciatica, Prostatic Hypertrophy, Recurrent Urinary Infections, Seborrhoea, Nephrotic Syndrome, Acne, Eyesight Problems, Heart Failure Hepatitis, Autism, Osteoporosis, Drug Addiction

Synopsis of integrative approach to health conditions and benefits 214

Impact of integration 220

Cost-benefit analysis 222

Summary 229

Glossary 233

Introduction

The human pursuit of health and longevity has taken many forms throughout history. From the ancient remedies utilized by early civilizations to the cutting-edge medical technology of the 21st century, our understanding of wellness and its various practices is both expansive and continually evolving.

In today's world, we have the privilege of choice. Modern or Western allopathic medicine offers scientifically validated treatments and quick relief for numerous ailments. However, people are increasingly turning to complementary and alternative therapies like yoga and Ayurveda, seeking holistic solutions to their health challenges.

The purpose of this book is to explore the benefits of combining modern medicine with yoga and Ayurveda, emphasizing their synergy in enhancing the overall health of individuals. This integrative approach acknowledges the strengths of each system and suggests that a combined effort can lead to more comprehensive health outcomes.

We begin by discussing the principles and practices of modern medicine. Known for its evidence-based treatments, modern medicine addresses symptoms of illness directly, often offering immediate relief. It excels in emergencies and the management of chronic conditions.

However, critics often point out that modern medicine tends to focus on the disease rather than the person. It sometimes overlooks the psychological and lifestyle aspects of health. Moreover, the side-effects of certain medications and treatments cannot be ignored.

Then we delve into yoga, a 5,000-year-old practice from India. Yoga goes beyond the physical postures (asanas) that most people associate with it. It includes ethical guidelines, breath control exercises, mindfulness practices, and meditation.

Regular yoga practice can help improve strength, flexibility, balance, and endurance. However, yoga's real power lies in its ability to promote mental well-being. It can reduce stress, improve concentration, and foster a sense of inner peace.

Next, we explore Ayurveda, an ancient holistic health care system also originating from India. Ayurveda focuses on maintaining a delicate balance between the mind, body, and spirit. It believes in the prevention of diseases through a balanced lifestyle, diet, and natural remedies.

Ayurveda sees every individual as unique, with a distinct body constitution (dosha). This understanding allows for personalized treatments, offering a different perspective on health compared to one-size-fits-all approaches.

Some critics argue that Ayurveda lacks scientific validation. However, an increasing number of research studies are demonstrating the effectiveness of various Ayurvedic practices, bringing a blend of tradition and science to health management.

The core of this book will examine the integration of modern medicine, yoga, and Ayurveda. Each of these systems has unique strengths. When combined, they can offer a multi-dimensional approach to health that is much more than the sum of its parts.

Modern medicine provides quick relief and robust solutions for acute conditions, while yoga offers a preventive approach that strengthens the body and calms the mind. Ayurveda, on the other hand, focuses on individualized wellness strategies based on a person's unique physical and mental constitution.

Together, they can address the physical, psychological, and lifestyle aspects of health, offering comprehensive care that can improve patient satisfaction and health outcomes.

This integration isn't about abandoning one system in favour of the other, but about finding balance. It's about choosing the best from each system based on the individual's unique needs, preferences, and circumstances.

The challenge of integrating these systems lies in reconciling their different philosophies, terminologies, and approaches. Yet, growing evidence suggests that this challenge is worth tackling, as the integration can result in enhanced health and well-being.

We'll share practical guidelines to seamlessly incorporate yoga and Ayurvedic principles into your life while continuing to benefit from the advancements of modern medicine. You'll learn how to communicate effectively with your healthcare providers about these practices and ensure they're part of your overall health strategy.

By embracing the concept of integrative health, we can begin to see health and wellness as a dynamic process that involves the interaction of mind, body, and spirit. This understanding can guide us towards more balanced, fulfilled, and healthy lives.

This book is not intended to replace the advice of medical professionals. Always consult with your healthcare provider before starting any new health regimen. The aim here is to broaden perspectives, presenting alternative approaches that can complement standard medical care.

The narrative ahead should serve as a compelling exploration of the untapped potential that lies in integrating modern medicine with yoga and Ayurveda. It's an invitation to view health from a wider perspective, one that acknowledges the complexity and uniqueness of the human being.

It is my hope that this book will not only educate you about the principles and practices of these health systems but also inspire you to implement this integrative approach in your life.

By merging the best of these worlds, we can harness the precision of modern medicine, the preventive and holistic nature of yoga, and the personalized wellness strategies of Ayurveda.

This blend of ancient wisdom and modern science can create a powerful tool for enhancing health and well-being.

It's time to shift the paradigm, to look beyond the confines of traditional methods, and to embrace a more comprehensive, inclusive approach to health care.

As we journey together through this exploration, it is my sincere belief that we'll unveil a richer understanding of health and well-being. One that highlights not just the absence of disease, but the presence of vitality, resilience, and joy.

This book is intended to be an engaging conversation, a meeting of minds, and an exploration of ideas. It's about broadening our horizons and discovering new paths towards optimal health.

I hope you find this blend of modern and ancient healing arts to be as fascinating as I do. It's a complex, dynamic, and ever-evolving field that offers immense potential for improving the quality of our lives.

Let's embark on this journey together. Let's discover how modern medicine, yoga, and Ayurveda can harmonize in a symphony of holistic health and wellness.

As we turn the page, let's keep an open mind and heart, ready to explore the transformative power that this integrative approach can bring to our lives.

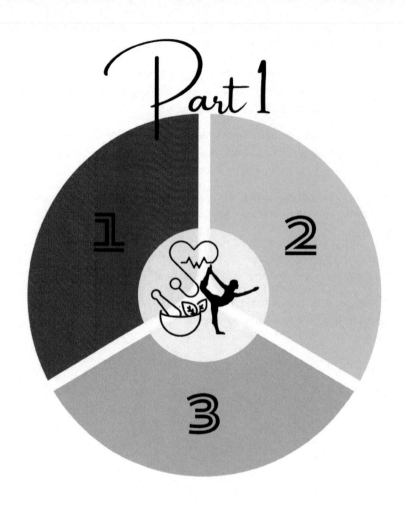

Part 1

Principles

VIEWING THE HEALTH FROM THE PERSPECTIVE OF MODERN MEDICINE, YOGA AND AYURVEDA

Identifying the differences and commonness to embark integration

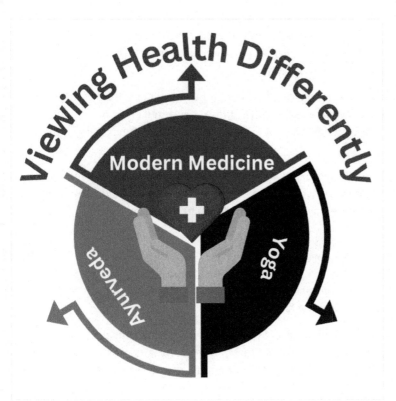

Defining Health from the Perspective of Modern Medicine

Modern medicine, often referred to as Western medicine or allopathic medicine, operates from a perspective that views health predominantly in physical terms. Health, in this model, is typically defined as the absence of disease or illness. This perspective has a strong focus on the body's biological systems and on identifying and treating symptoms of illness.

Diagnosis and treatment in modern medicine often involve the use of clinical examination, investigations, use of pharmaceuticals, surgery, and other interventions designed to restore the body's normal function. Health is, therefore, seen as achieving and maintaining normal physiological function, with the body's various systems operating smoothly and effectively.

In this view, a person is healthy if they do not exhibit signs of disease, their vital signs are within an acceptable range, their body functions normally, and they can carry out their daily activities without undue fatigue or physical stress. This medical model is particularly effective in handling acute and life-threatening illnesses and conditions.

Understanding Modern Medicine

The Modern medicine represents a fundamental pillar in our global healthcare system. Developed through rigorous scientific research and clinical trials, it provides a wide array of effective treatments for many acute and chronic conditions.

Its focus on disease pathology, coupled with the rapid advancements in technology, has led to ground-breaking medical discoveries and innovations. From life-saving surgeries and powerful pharmaceuticals to advanced diagnostic techniques, modern medicine excels at treating symptoms directly and often rapidly.

The field of modern medicine is expansive. It covers various specialties, from cardiology and neurology to psychiatry and orthopaedics. Each of these specialized areas offers specific treatments for the associated conditions, contributing to the holistic functioning of the medical field.

The progress made in modern medicine has undeniably extended our lifespan and improved our quality of life. Countless lives have been saved through emergency medical procedures, and many chronic conditions are now manageable thanks to the development of advanced drugs.

However, modern medicine is not without its challenges. Critics argue that it often employs a reductionist approach, treating the body as a machine composed of individual parts rather than an interconnected whole. This perspective can lead to treatments that address the symptoms of a disease without getting to the root cause.

Additionally, while the advent of pharmaceuticals has been a game-changer in disease management, concerns about the overuse of drugs and the associated side effects have been raised. Some medications, while alleviating symptoms, can lead to other health issues or dependencies.

Despite these criticisms, the role of modern medicine in healthcare is irreplaceable. Its strength in diagnosing and treating disease, especially in acute and emergency situations, is unparalleled. It's a crucial component in our collective health and wellbeing.

Modern medicine thus presents a very specific perspective on health. Its central focus is on the physical body and its functioning, with the primary goal being to cure disease and alleviate symptoms. In the modern medical model, health is often seen as a state of being free from illness or disease. A person is typically considered healthy if they do not exhibit physical signs of disease or dysfunction. "This medical model is particularly effective in handling acute and life-threatening illnesses and conditions."

Modern medicine model emphasizes the importance of regular check-ups and screenings to identify and address potential health issues as early as possible. The objective is to detect signs of disease or abnormality and intervene before these progress into more serious health problems.

"Modern medicine places a high emphasis on evidence-based practice and scientific research". Diseases are classified based on their symptoms and the organs they affect, and treatments are chosen based on the effectiveness demonstrated in clinical trials.

A central principle of modern medicine is the concept of homeostasis – the body's ability to maintain a stable internal environment in response to changes in external conditions. Health, therefore, is seen as the body's ability to maintain this balance and effectively respond to changes and challenges.

In this framework, each part of the body is often seen in isolation, and diseases are often treated by specialists who focus on a particular organ or system. This approach has led to significant advancements in the understanding and treatment of specific diseases.

In modern medicine, technology plays a crucial role in defining and diagnosing health. Advanced diagnostic tools like MRI, CT scans, and blood tests allow for a detailed analysis of the body's functioning, helping to identify signs of disease or dysfunction.

The success of modern medicine lies in its ability to treat acute illnesses and life-threatening conditions effectively. It excels in situations where immediate medical intervention is necessary, such as surgery or the use of life-saving medications.

However, the modern medical model has been criticized for its disease-centric approach, which tends to focus more on treating symptoms rather than addressing underlying causes. Critics argue that it often overlooks the importance of lifestyle factors in health and well-being.

Furthermore, critics argue that the modern medical model often neglects the emotional and psychological dimensions of health. While it is effective at treating physical symptoms, it may not always address the mental and emotional aspects that are integral to overall well-being.

Modern medicine's biomedical model views health is largely followed across the world and is a physical phenomenon, with disease considered a deviation from the norm of bodily function. This model promotes a systemic approach, often treating the body as a machine composed of different parts that can be treated separately.

The advancement of technology has played a significant role in shaping the modern medical perspective. The ability to detect, diagnose, and treat illnesses has seen a remarkable improvement due to advancements like imaging techniques, laboratory tests, and pharmaceutical interventions.

Allopathic medicine relies heavily on evidence-based practice, utilizing rigorous scientific research to establish the most effective treatment methods. This brings a sense of certainty and predictability in the treatment outcomes of many health conditions.

The disease-focused approach of modern medicine, while critical for treating acute and life-threatening conditions, can sometimes overlook the importance of prevention and health promotion. Lifestyle diseases, such as heart disease and type 2 diabetes, are increasingly prevalent, demanding a broader view of health.

Despite some criticisms, modern medicine has significantly contributed to improving human health, particularly in managing infectious diseases, surgical procedures, and emergency care. Its power lies in its ability to address immediate health crises and its commitment to continuous scientific advancements.

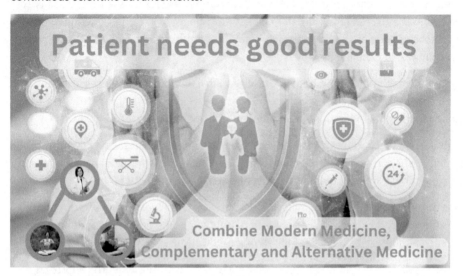

Understanding Health from perspective of Yoga

As we shift our focus from modern medicine, we venture into the world of yoga, an ancient practice that originated in India over 5000 years ago. Yoga is a comprehensive wellness regimen that incorporates physical postures (asanas), breathing techniques (pranayama), and meditation (dhyana).

Yoga is more than just a form of exercise. It is a mind-body practice that seeks to harmonize the individual with the self, the world, and the divine. Its ultimate goal is not just physical fitness, but spiritual enlightenment and self-realization.

Regular yoga practice offers a wealth of health benefits. On the physical level, yoga can increase flexibility, build strength, improve balance, enhance cardiovascular health, and promote healthy weight.

However, yoga's power extends far beyond physical health. It's particularly renowned for its effects on mental wellbeing. Regular practice can reduce stress, improve concentration, promote better sleep, increase body awareness, and foster a sense of inner peace and contentment.

Recent scientific research supports these benefits. Numerous studies have highlighted yoga's role in reducing anxiety and depression, managing stress, improving cognitive function, and enhancing overall quality of life.

Yoga also emphasizes mindfulness and the cultivation of a positive mind-body relationship. Through the practice, individuals learn to tune into their bodies, to respect their boundaries, and to understand the interconnection between physical health and mental wellbeing.

Despite the increasing popularity of yoga in the Western world, some misconceptions persist. Yoga is not just for the flexible or the fit; it can be adapted to suit all fitness levels and ages. It's also not a religion, but a philosophy that promotes harmony and balance.

Through regular practice, yoga can be an empowering tool, fostering self-care and promoting overall health and wellbeing. By combining asanas, pranayama, and dhyana, individuals can cultivate a holistic sense of wellness that permeates all aspects of their lives.

Understanding Health from the Perspective of Yoga

Yoga, with its roots in ancient Indian philosophy, presents a more holistic definition of health. It doesn't view health merely as the absence of disease but as a state of complete physical, mental, and spiritual well-being.

The practice of yoga includes physical postures (asanas), breathing techniques (pranayama), and meditation (dhyana), all of which work together to bring harmony to the body, mind, and spirit. Therefore, health in yoga is not only about physical fitness but also about cultivating a calm mind and a harmonious state of being.

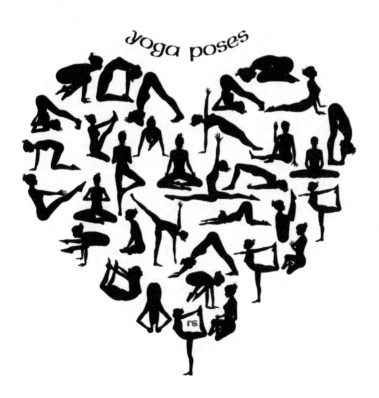

yoga poses

According to yoga philosophy, health is a balanced state where the body is strong and flexible, the mind is calm and clear, and the individual is connected to a deeper sense of self and purpose. It acknowledges the interconnectedness of the physical, emotional, and spiritual dimensions of our being.

Thus the perspective on health from yoga, differs significantly from that of modern medicine. Yoga views health in a more holistic manner, incorporating physical, mental, and spiritual dimensions.

In yoga, health is not just seen as freedom from disease. Instead, it is a state of holistic well-being, where the body is strong, the mind is clear, and the individual is in harmony with themselves and their environment.

Yoga believes that true health involves balance. This balance relates not just to physical well-being but also to mental and spiritual harmony. A person is considered healthy if they maintain a balance between their physical, mental, and spiritual selves.

The elements of yoga i.e. physical postures (asanas), breath control (pranayama), and meditation (dhyana) work together to promote physical health, calm the mind, and help the practitioner achieve a deeper state of consciousness.

In yoga, physical health is important but not the only focus. A healthy body is seen as a vessel that supports the individual in achieving a higher state of consciousness. As such, physical postures in yoga are often used as a tool to prepare the body for meditation.

Yoga considers mental health to be equally important as physical health. It emphasizes the role of mindfulness and self-awareness in maintaining mental well-being. A regular yoga practice can help manage stress, enhance concentration, and promote a positive mental state.

From a yoga perspective, spiritual health is a crucial aspect of overall well-being. Spirituality is not tied to any particular religion or belief system. Instead, it refers to the recognition of a sense of connectedness with all living beings and the universe as a whole.

Yoga views health as a lifelong journey, not a destination. It encourages the practitioner to cultivate a holistic lifestyle that includes a balanced diet, regular exercise, adequate sleep, and a positive mind-set.

Critics of yoga argue that while it offers significant benefits, it cannot replace modern medicine in treating acute illnesses or severe medical conditions. However, most people recognize that it as a valuable complementary practice that can improve overall health and quality of life.

Ultimately, yoga offers a unique perspective on health, emphasizing the interconnection between the body, mind, and spirit. It provides a wealth of practices and philosophies that can enhance well-being and contribute to a holistic understanding of health.

In contrast to western medicine, yoga provides a more comprehensive and interconnected perspective on health. Rooted in ancient wisdom, it aims to harmonize the body, mind, and spirit, promoting holistic health and wellness.

Yoga, which means "to yoke" or "unite," sees health as a state of unity within oneself and with the external world. It acknowledges the intricate relationship between our physical health and our thoughts, emotions, and consciousness.

The yogic view of health goes beyond mere physical wellness. It includes mental clarity, emotional stability, self-awareness, and a sense of inner peace. The practice of yoga, through asanas, pranayama, and meditation, serves as a tool to achieve this balance.

Yoga encourages self-exploration and self-care. It promotes a proactive approach to health, where maintaining balance and harmony is key. A regular yoga practice can lead to improved physical health, stress management, and spiritual growth.

The growing recognition of yoga's health benefits has led to its integration with modern healthcare. While not a replacement for medical treatment, yoga can complement it by enhancing overall wellbeing, promoting recovery, and improving quality of life.

Yoga, unlike modern medicine, is founded on the principles of unity and balance. It recognizes the interconnectedness of the mind, body, and spirit and aims to bring them into harmony.

The principle of self-awareness is key in yoga. Through various practices such as asanas (postures), pranayama (breathing techniques), and dhyana (meditation), yoga encourages practitioners to cultivate mindfulness and awareness of their inner states.

Another principle of yoga is Ahimsa, or non-violence. This includes not causing harm to oneself or others, both physically and mentally. This principle is often applied in the practice of yoga through a respectful and mindful approach to one's body and capabilities.

Yoga also emphasizes the principle of Svadhyaya, or self-study. This involves self-reflection and introspection to gain self-knowledge and understanding.

Additionally, yoga advocates for a healthy lifestyle. This includes a balanced diet, regular physical activity, and mental practices for stress management and inner peace.

Understanding Ayurveda: The Ancient Art of Healing

As we delve deeper into the realm of holistic health practices, we encounter Ayurveda. Translated as the "science of life," Ayurveda is one of the oldest holistic healing systems in the world, with roots in ancient India.

At its core, Ayurveda is based on the principle that health and wellness depend on a delicate balance between the mind, body, and spirit. It sees the individual as an integral part of the universe, interconnected and affected by its elements.

Unlike modern medicine, which focuses primarily on treating disease, Ayurveda prioritizes prevention. It encourages the maintenance of health through close attention to balance in one's life, right thinking, diet, lifestyle, and the use of herbs.

According to Ayurveda, each person is a unique combination of the five universal elements: space, air, fire, water, and earth. These elements combine to form three life forces or energies, known as doshas: Vata, Pitta, and Kapha. Every individual has a unique balance of these doshas, defining their physical and mental characteristics.

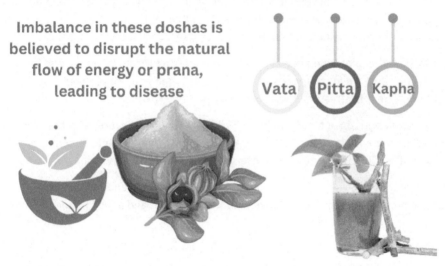

Imbalance in these doshas is believed to disrupt the natural flow of energy or prana, leading to disease

Vata Pitta Kapha

An imbalance in these doshas is believed to disrupt the natural flow of energy, or prana, leading to disease. Ayurveda's goal is to restore this balance, often through natural remedies, dietary changes, and lifestyle adjustments.

Despite being thousands of years old, Ayurveda remains relevant today. Its focus on personalized treatment and its holistic approach have gained recognition in the global health community. It's particularly appreciated for its focus on wellness, which encompasses not just the absence of illness but the presence of positive vitality.

Critics often argue that Ayurveda lacks scientific validation. However, an increasing number of studies are providing evidence for the efficacy of various Ayurvedic practices and treatments. Moreover, Ayurveda's emphasis on preventative healthcare and personalized treatment resonates strongly with contemporary understanding of chronic disease management and wellness.

It's essential to note that while Ayurveda offers extensive wisdom about health and wellness, it doesn't replace the need for modern medical treatment. Instead, it complements it, offering strategies for disease prevention, overall health improvement, and lifestyle management.

Defining Health from the Perspective of Ayurveda

Ayurveda, another ancient Indian science of life and health, also proposes a holistic definition of health. Its approach goes beyond the physical body to include the mind, spirit, senses, and relationships with others and with the natural world.

In Ayurveda, health is not just the absence of disease, but a state of balance. This balance is understood in terms of three fundamental energies or "doshas" – Vata, Pitta, and Kapha – which govern the body's physiological activity. A person is considered healthy when these doshas are in equilibrium, the digestive fire (Agni) is in a balanced state, the bodily tissues and functions are working efficiently, and the soul, senses, and mind are in a state of contentment and peace.

In this view, optimal health is achieved through a balanced lifestyle that nurtures the body, mind, and spirit. This includes proper diet, exercise, self-care practices, and a harmonious relationship with nature and society.

Each person is born with a unique balance of these doshas, known as their constitution or "prakriti". Health is maintaining the balance of doshas according to one's prakriti. Disease or ill-health is considered to be a state of imbalance, or "vikriti".

Ayurveda emphasizes the importance of "Agni" or digestive fire. A balanced Agni is key to good health as it ensures proper digestion and absorption of nutrients, and efficient elimination of waste products.

Ayurveda takes into account the whole individual—body, mind, and spirit—in the process of diagnosis and treatment. It emphasizes the connection between the individual and their environment, and the influence of lifestyle and dietary habits on health.

In Ayurveda, mental and emotional health are seen as crucial to overall well-being. The concept of "sattva" (mental clarity or purity) is considered important for maintaining mental and emotional balance.

Ayurveda recommends a variety of lifestyle practices for maintaining health and preventing disease. These include a balanced diet, regular physical activity, adequate rest, and practices for mental and spiritual well-being such as meditation and yoga.

Herbs and natural substances play a key role in Ayurvedic medicine as therapeutic agents. They are used not only for treating disease but also for promoting health and longevity.

Ayurveda also values the concept of "swasthavritta" or personal hygiene, both internal and external, as a means of maintaining health. This includes not only physical cleanliness but also cleanliness of the mind and spirit.

While Ayurveda offers a detailed and holistic approach to health, critics argue that it lacks the empirical evidence and research base of modern medicine. However, an increasing number of scientific studies are exploring the efficacy of Ayurvedic practices and treatments, validating its contributions to health and wellness.

Ayurveda also values emotional and spiritual health. It underscores the importance of positive relationships, ethical living, and connection with nature as part of a healthy lifestyle.

Despite Ayurveda's comprehensive view of health, it is often criticized for its lack of empirical evidence. However, the increasing scientific investigation of Ayurvedic principles and treatments is beginning to validate its effectiveness and its potential for integration with modern healthcare.

The Harmony of Modern Medicine, Yoga and Ayurveda

Having explored the principles of modern medicine, yoga, and Ayurveda, we now turn our attention to how these systems can work together. Each of these practices, with their unique perspectives and methodologies, brings something different to the healthcare table.

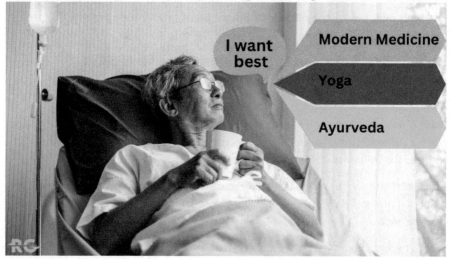

Modern medicine excels at diagnosing and treating acute conditions and managing chronic diseases. It offers powerful tools for rapid symptom relief and lifesaving interventions. Its strength lies in its scientific rigor, its ability to standardize treatments, and its focus on disease pathology.

On the other hand, yoga offers a preventive approach to health, with physical, mental, and spiritual benefits. It can strengthen the body, calm the mind, and instil a sense of inner peace and balance. Its emphasis on mindfulness and self-care empowers individuals to play an active role in their health.

Ayurveda, with its holistic and individual-centric view of health, offers personalized wellness strategies. Its focus on balancing the mind, body, and spirit, and its preventive approach, aligns well with contemporary understanding of wellness and chronic disease management.

Together, these systems can offer a multi-dimensional approach to health, providing comprehensive care that improves patient outcomes and satisfaction. By acknowledging and integrating the strengths of each system, we can move towards a model of health that is person-centred, holistic, and empowering.

The goal of this integrated approach is not to replace one system with another but to find the most effective combination for each individual. It's about respecting the uniqueness of each person, their health condition, and their personal beliefs and preferences.

The beauty of this integration lies in its flexibility and adaptability. It can be tailored to meet the unique needs and preferences of each individual. This personalized approach not only improves health outcomes but also enhances the individual's engagement and satisfaction with their healthcare.

Integrating modern medicine with yoga and Ayurveda doesn't mean disregarding the science that underpins modern healthcare. Instead, it invites us to expand our understanding of health, to include not just the physical but also the mental, emotional, and spiritual dimensions.

As we continue on this journey, we'll explore this integrated approach further, delving into practical guidelines, real-life case studies, and scientific evidence. The goal is to provide a comprehensive understanding of how these systems can work together to promote optimal health and wellness.

It's important to note that while this integrated approach offers many benefits, it's not a magic bullet. Just like any other healthcare approach, it requires commitment, consistency, and patience. Moreover, it should be guided by qualified healthcare professionals to ensure safety and effectiveness.

The path towards optimal health is a personal journey, one that is unique to each of us. By combining the best of modern medicine, yoga, and Ayurveda, we can empower ourselves to navigate this journey with wisdom, balance, and resilience. Together, these practices can light the way towards a more holistic, integrative understanding of health and wellbeing.

Practical Implementation of an Integrative Approach

How can we implement this integrative approach to health in our lives? This chapter offers some guidance on how to incorporate the principles and practices of yoga and Ayurveda into your life while continuing to benefit from the advancements of modern medicine.

If you feel comfortable, begin by consulting with your healthcare providers. Talk to them about your interest in yoga and Ayurveda, and discuss how these practices might fit into your current health plan. They can guide you on how to safely incorporate these practices and may also provide referrals to qualified practitioners.

When starting with yoga, consider joining a class or working with a certified yoga instructor. They can guide you through the correct postures, help you modify poses based on your fitness level, and ensure your practice is safe and beneficial.

Starting slow is key. Yoga is not about being the most flexible or executing the most challenging poses; it's about connecting with your body and mind. Allow your body time to adjust to the new movements. As your strength and flexibility increase, your yoga practice can become more challenging and diverse.

Mindfulness is a core aspect of yoga. Try to incorporate mindfulness into your practice by focusing on your breath, being aware of how your body feels, and cultivating a sense of inner peace and relaxation.

If you're interested in Ayurveda, consider consulting with an Ayurvedic practitioner. They can help determine your dosha, provide personalized recommendations for diet and lifestyle, and guide you on using Ayurvedic remedies.

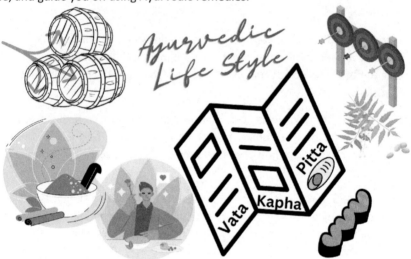

Ayurveda places a strong emphasis on diet. Eating a balanced, nutritious diet tailored to your dosha can help maintain balance and health. Regular exercise, adequate sleep, and stress management techniques are also vital components of an Ayurvedic lifestyle.

Integrating modern medicine, yoga, and Ayurveda requires open communication among all your healthcare providers. Ensure each is aware of the treatments and practices you are using. This can help prevent potential interactions and ensure all your health needs are being addressed.

Remember, this integrated approach is not about replacing one system with another; it's about using the best that each has to offer. It's about creating a personalized health plan that addresses your unique needs and promotes your overall wellbeing.

Practical examples for integrated approach

The principle of integrated medicine—bridging modern, Ayurvedic, and Yoga interventions—has indeed shown its potential across a spectrum of health issues. Considering these therapies as complementary, rather than exclusive, opens avenues for broader, more holistic patient care, encompassing physical, mental, and emotional dimensions of health.

Consider the chronic problem of insomnia, which often intertwines with other physical and mental health issues. While modern medicine may prescribe sedatives or behaviour therapy, Ayurveda emphasizes on balancing the body's doshas and improving sleep hygiene through dietary and lifestyle changes. Yoga can complement these strategies with practices like Yoga Nidra and meditation that calm the mind and prepare the body for restful sleep.

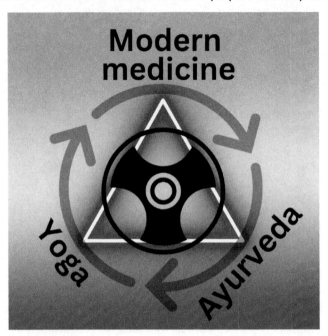

Anorexia nervosa, an eating disorder marked by an intense fear of gaining weight, can similarly benefit from a comprehensive approach. Modern medicine addresses the issue with medications and cognitive behavioural therapy. Ayurveda recommends a balanced diet, specific herbs, and procedures to improve digestion and stimulate appetite, while yoga's mindfulness-based practices can help individuals rebuild a healthier relationship with food and body image.

Allergies, often due to hyperactive immune system, can be managed with a combination of antihistamines and immunotherapy from modern medicine, immune-modulating herbs from Ayurveda, and yoga practices that help manage stress and maintain respiratory health.

Alzheimer's disease and Parkinson's disease, degenerative neurological disorders, could also be addressed in this integrated framework. While modern medicine aims to slow disease progression and manage symptoms, Ayurveda and yoga may help improve overall mental function, stress management, balance, and coordination.

Sciatica and prostatic hypertrophy, painful conditions affecting the back and prostate gland respectively, can be managed with pain relief medications and surgery in severe cases. Ayurvedic herbs and oils can reduce inflammation, while specific yoga poses can enhance blood flow, flexibility, and strength in the affected areas.

The approach is equally useful in addressing frequent urinary tract infections, seborrhoea, and nephrotic syndrome. While modern medicine offers antibiotics and other drugs to control these conditions, Ayurveda and yoga can support overall urinary and skin health, and boost immunity.

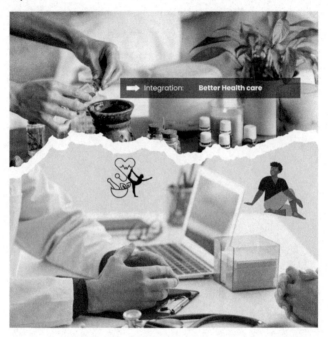

Thus the amalgamation of modern medicine, Ayurveda, and yoga appears promising in addressing numerous health conditions. By complementing each other's strengths, these systems work synergistically, potentially leading to better outcomes. They offer an inclusive health strategy, addressing the root cause of diseases, rather than just treating symptoms, promoting not just the absence of disease, but the presence of health. Some more examples of the integration of modern, Ayurvedic, and Yoga therapies also reinforce the integration as a potent strategy for managing more prevalent health concerns.

Acne, a common skin issue caused due to sebum and dead skin cell accumulation in hair follicles, is typically treated with topical or oral medication in modern medicine. Ayurveda, on the other hand, recommends detoxification, along with specific herbs to balance doshas and improve skin health. Yoga, with its focus on improving circulation and reducing stress, could be instrumental in managing acne as well.

Eye sight problems, like myopia and hypermetropia, are usually corrected with glasses, contact lenses, or surgical procedures in modern medicine. However, Ayurvedic treatments such as Netra Tarpana can nourish and rejuvenate the eyes, while specific Yoga exercises, like Tratak, could help enhance visual concentration and relax ocular muscles.

Heart failure, a serious condition where the heart can't pump blood efficiently, is typically managed with medications, lifestyle changes, and potentially surgery in modern medicine.

Ayurveda may support cardiac function and circulation through herbs like Arjuna, while Yoga could aid in stress management and improving physical stamina.

Hepatitis, an inflammation of the liver, is treated with antiviral drugs in modern medicine, while Ayurveda uses herbs and detox procedures to support liver function and overall immunity. Yoga asanas, especially those that stimulate the abdominal region, could be beneficial in promoting liver health.

Autism, a neurodevelopmental disorder, is managed with behavioural and communication therapies in modern medicine. Ayurveda employs a holistic approach, using specific herbs to balance brain function, while Yoga's structured, calming practices may improve focus and behaviour in autistic individuals.

Osteoporosis, a bone weakening condition, is generally treated with medications and supplements to improve bone density in modern medicine. Ayurveda focuses on nutrition, herbs, and therapies for bone strength, while weight-bearing Yoga asanas could help improve bone density and balance.

In managing drug addiction, modern medicine provides medications to manage withdrawal symptoms and prevent relapse. Ayurveda employs detoxification procedures and rejuvenating herbs to restore body balance, while Yoga's mindfulness and self-awareness practices can help individuals break the cycle of addiction.

In conclusion, blending modern, Ayurvedic, and Yoga therapies provides a comprehensive, multi-dimensional approach to health and wellness. By capitalizing on the strengths of each practice, this integrative approach can enhance patient care, contributing to overall well-being and an improved quality of life.

Commonness in principles of modern medicine, yoga and Ayurveda

While modern medicine, yoga, and Ayurveda each have their own unique principles, there are several common threads that run through all three.

One such principle is the recognition of the holistic nature of health. All three acknowledge that health is more than just the absence of disease, and involves the complete physical, mental, emotional, and social well-being of an individual.

The principle of prevention is another commonality. Modern medicine, through vaccinations and health screenings, yoga, through balance and mindfulness, and Ayurveda, through balanced doshas and Agni, all emphasize the importance of preventing disease before it occurs.

The idea of balance also resonates across all three. In modern medicine, it may refer to the balance of different bodily systems. In yoga, it's about the balance between the mind, body, and spirit, and in Ayurveda, it pertains to the balance of the doshas.

Respect for the individual's autonomy is also a shared principle. Modern medicine respects patient autonomy through informed consent, yoga encourages self-awareness and self-care, and Ayurveda recognizes individual uniqueness through the concept of Prakriti.

All three also place value on the importance of lifestyle in health. Whether it's through diet, physical activity, stress management, or mental practices, all three recognize that lifestyle choices play a significant role in health and well-being.

Despite the differences in their origins and approaches, the principles of modern medicine, yoga, and Ayurveda show remarkable alignment. Each of these systems offers valuable insights into health and well-being, and their shared principles provide a foundation for an integrated approach to health.

Recognizing these common principles can facilitate a deeper understanding of health. It can help us see beyond the narrow lens of disease and appreciate health as a dynamic state of complete well-being.

This recognition can also encourage a more comprehensive approach to healthcare. By integrating the strengths of modern medicine, yoga, and Ayurveda, we can address not just the physical aspects of health, but also the mental, emotional, and social dimensions.

Finally, understanding these common principles can empower individuals to take charge of their health. It can inspire them to make healthier lifestyle choices, seek preventive measures, respect their unique needs and capacities, and strive for a state of balance and holistic well-being.

It is also important to note that while these principles may align, their applications may differ across these systems. The key is to find the right balance and integration that works for the individual.

The intersection of these principles forms a compelling vision of health, one that is holistic, preventative, balanced, respectful of individual autonomy, and recognizes the importance of lifestyle. This vision can guide us towards a healthcare system that is not just about treating diseases, but about promoting overall well-being.

By embracing these common principles, we have the opportunity to transform our understanding of health and our approach to healthcare. We can move towards a system that values and promotes overall well-being, where individuals are empowered to be active participants in their health, and where healthcare providers are facilitators of holistic health.

With an integrated approach, we can harness the strengths of modern medicine, yoga, and Ayurveda, bringing together the best of all worlds for the benefit of individual and public health.

Ultimately, the goal of health, as seen through the lens of these common principles, is not just to live, but to live well. It's about cultivating a state of complete physical, mental, and social well-being, and leading a life of balance, fulfilment, and purpose.

Harmonising the Three Perspectives MYA – Modern medicine, Yoga and Ayurveda

These definitions of health from modern medicine, yoga, and Ayurveda each offer valuable perspectives. Modern medicine excels at diagnosing and treating disease, particularly acute and severe conditions. Yoga offers valuable tools for promoting physical health, mental clarity, and spiritual growth. Ayurveda provides a comprehensive approach to lifestyle, diet, and herbal remedies that aim to prevent disease and promote overall wellbeing.

The integration of these three perspectives can provide a more holistic and comprehensive approach to health. Modern medicine provides a powerful tool for managing disease and health crises. Yoga offers a wealth of practices for maintaining physical health, managing stress, and promoting mental and emotional wellbeing. Ayurveda offers practical guidance on diet, lifestyle, and natural remedies that can help prevent disease and promote optimal health.

Integrating these perspectives means recognizing that health is more than the absence of disease. It is a dynamic state of balance and wellbeing that encompasses the whole person – body, mind, and spirit.

From this integrated perspective, health involves maintaining physical fitness and normal physiological function (modern medicine), nurturing mental clarity and emotional wellbeing (yoga), and cultivating a balanced lifestyle that supports our unique constitution (Ayurveda).

In this holistic view, health is not a static state but a dynamic process. It involves ongoing care and attention to our physical, mental, and emotional wellbeing. It requires us to be active participants in our health, making choices that support our wellbeing and align with our unique needs and life circumstances.

This integrated view of health empowers us to take charge of our health and wellbeing. It encourages us to view health as an investment, not just a goal. And it offers us a rich array of tools and strategies – from modern medicine, yoga, and Ayurveda – that we can use to enhance our health and wellbeing.

This integrated perspective also recognizes the influence of our environment and lifestyle on our health. It acknowledges that our health is impacted by the quality of our relationships, the food we eat, the way we handle stress, and our connection with nature and the world around us.

Embracing an integrative approach to health means recognizing the value of each perspective and drawing on the strengths of modern medicine, yoga, and Ayurveda. It means taking a proactive approach to our health, focusing on prevention and wellness, not just disease and treatment.

It means respecting our body's innate healing wisdom, nurturing our mental and emotional wellbeing, and cultivating a lifestyle that supports balance and vitality. And most importantly, it means honouring our unique health journey, recognizing that each of us is unique and that what works best for one person may not work for another.

As we look to the future of health and wellness, this integrated perspective holds great promise. It invites us to redefine health in a more holistic and person-centred way. And it offers us the tools and strategies we need to thrive – not just physically, but also mentally and spiritually.

In closing, the definitions of health provided by modern medicine, yoga, and Ayurveda, while seemingly different, can indeed be harmonious. By considering health holistically and integrating the best of these three health modalities, we can all work towards achieving and maintaining a truly balanced state of health.

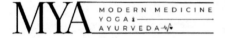

Addressing concerns in Integrating Modern Medicine, Yoga, and Ayurveda (MYA)

The perspectives of modern medicine, yoga, and Ayurveda on health, while different, are not mutually exclusive. Each offers unique insights and approaches that can contribute to a more comprehensive understanding of health.

Modern medicine provides a detailed understanding of the body's structure and function, and effective treatments for a wide range of diseases. Yoga offers practices for physical health and techniques for managing stress and enhancing mental and emotional well-being. Ayurveda provides a holistic approach to health and wellness, focusing on diet, lifestyle, and the balance of bio-energies.

Each of these three systems of health – modern medicine, yoga, and Ayurveda thus provides valuable insights and approaches that can contribute to a more holistic understanding and management of health.

Modern medicine offers effective treatment modalities for acute conditions and life-threatening diseases, yoga aids in the harmonization of body, mind, and spirit, and Ayurveda offers a holistic health system focusing on the balance of body's energies and lifestyle modifications.

By integrating these perspectives, we can address health from a more holistic standpoint. This involves not only treating disease but also promoting overall well-being—physically, mentally, and spiritually.

An integrated approach can help us recognize the interconnectedness of different aspects of our health. For instance, how our mental state can affect our physical health, or how our lifestyle and diet can impact our overall well-being.

This approach allows us to draw on a wider range of tools and strategies for maintaining health and treating disease. From modern medicine, we can avail of cutting-edge treatments and diagnostics. From yoga, we can learn practices for physical health and mental balance. And from Ayurveda, we can gain insights into diet, lifestyle, and natural remedies.

This integrated approach to health does not mean disregarding the benefits and effectiveness of modern medicine. Instead, it means complementing it with other health practices that focus on prevention and enhancing overall well-being.

It encourages us to be active participants in our health, taking care of our physical well-being, cultivating a positive mental state, and leading a balanced lifestyle.

An integrative perspective on health recognizes that each individual is unique. What works for one person may not work for another. Therefore, it allows for personalized health strategies that take into account an individual's physical constitution, mental state, lifestyle, and personal preferences.

In this way, an integrative approach to health goes beyond merely treating disease. It promotes a culture of health, where the focus is not just on living disease-free, but on living well.

Furthermore, defining health from the perspectives of modern medicine, yoga, and Ayurveda allows us to appreciate the complexity and interconnectedness of health. While each offers a distinct viewpoint, together they provide a richer and more holistic understanding of what it means to be truly healthy. It invites us to explore new possibilities for health and well-being, drawing on the best of what each has to offer.

Integrating these three systems could potentially bring a more comprehensive, personalized, and preventive approach to health and wellness. It promotes a model of health that values both disease management and the promotion of wellbeing, taking into consideration the physical, mental, and spiritual dimensions of health.

It's also about understanding that one size does not fit all when it comes to health. What works for one person may not work for another. An integrative approach provides a broader toolkit and respects individual preferences and needs.

Despite their differences, modern medicine, yoga, and Ayurveda share a common goal: to promote health and wellbeing. By integrating their strengths, we can work towards a more holistic, person-centred healthcare that doesn't just focus on treating diseases but also on promoting overall wellbeing. The integration of these practices invites us to reimagine health in its fullest sense - as a state of complete physical, mental, and social wellbeing.

Benefits of integration of Modern Medicine, Yoga, and Ayurveda (MYA)

The strength of modern medicine is well-established, with its precise diagnostic tools, powerful drugs, and sophisticated surgeries. However, it's increasingly recognized that this approach can sometimes be reductionist, focusing on specific diseases and symptoms without always considering the broader context of an individual's health and lifestyle. That's where yoga and Ayurveda, ancient systems of well-being, come in. When combined, these three offer an integrative, holistic approach to health that can not only treat diseases but also promote wellness and prevent future health issues.

Cardiovascular health is a global concern with heart disease being a leading cause of death. Modern medicine offers various interventions like statins for cholesterol management, antihypertensives, and surgeries. However, these don't address underlying lifestyle factors that often drive these diseases. Yoga, with its emphasis on physical activity and stress reduction, has been shown to improve cardiovascular health. Ayurveda, through dietary recommendations and natural remedies, also supports heart health. Combining these with modern treatments can provide a more comprehensive approach to cardiovascular care.

Respiratory disorders like asthma and COPD can significantly affect a person's quality of life. While modern medicine provides drugs to manage symptoms, yoga offers breathing techniques that improve lung capacity and function. Ayurveda can help identify and mitigate dietary and environmental triggers of respiratory issues. Together, these three approaches can help patients manage symptoms more effectively.

Neurological disorders such as Parkinson's, Alzheimer's, and multiple sclerosis pose significant challenges for modern medicine due to their complex nature. Yoga's focus on mindfulness and physical stability can enhance mental health and mobility, while Ayurvedic practices can support overall neurological health. When combined with conventional treatments, these can enhance quality of life for those with neurological conditions.

Digestive disorders can be deeply affected by diet and lifestyle, areas often addressed inadequately by modern medicine. Ayurveda, with its emphasis on healthy dietary practices, can provide natural remedies and personalized diet plans, while yoga can improve digestion through physical postures. This integrative approach can offer a more holistic treatment for digestive disorders.

Endocrine disorders like diabetes and thyroid disorders are rising globally. Modern medicine offers hormone replacement therapy and other treatments, but these often have side effects. Yoga, through its stress-reducing and hormone-regulating effects, can support endocrine health. Ayurveda provides dietary and herbal solutions for these disorders. Integrating these with modern medicine can result in more comprehensive and effective care.

For reproductive health, the combination of modern medicine, yoga, and Ayurveda is promising. While modern medicine provides hormonal treatments and surgeries, yoga can enhance fertility and sexual health through specific postures and stress reduction. Ayurveda's emphasis on diet and lifestyle can improve reproductive health and fertility. This integrated approach can provide a well-rounded treatment strategy for both male and female reproductive issues.

Skin disorders like eczema, psoriasis, and acne often require long-term management. Modern medicine offers topical and systemic treatments, but these can have side effects. Yoga's stress-reducing effects can benefit skin health, and Ayurveda offers dietary advice and natural remedies. An integrated approach can provide a more holistic and sustainable solution for skin disorders.

Haematological conditions like anaemia and clotting disorders can be life-altering. Modern medicine provides blood transfusions and drugs, but these can have side effects and don't always address underlying issues. Yoga can improve circulation, and Ayurveda can offer dietary advice to support blood health. An integrative approach can offer a broader solution for these disorders.

Infectious diseases and immune disorders pose a significant challenge for modern medicine. While antibiotics and other drugs are critical, they don't support the immune system. Yoga's stress-reducing and immune-enhancing benefits can support immune health, and Ayurveda offers dietary and herbal interventions to enhance immunity. Combining these with modern treatments can offer a more comprehensive approach to infectious and immune conditions.

Lastly, reproductive problems like infertility, menstrual disorders, and menopausal symptoms can be complex. Modern medicine offers hormonal therapies and assisted reproductive technologies, but these can be invasive and have side effects. Yoga can support reproductive health through stress reduction and hormone balance, and Ayurveda offers dietary and lifestyle interventions. An integrated approach can provide a more personalized and holistic treatment for these problems.

The combination of modern medicine, yoga, and Ayurveda for disease treatment and prevention offers a patient-centered, comprehensive approach. It combines the best of scientific advances with ancient wisdom, addressing not just the disease but the whole person. It has the potential to improve health outcomes, patient satisfaction, and overall health care.

However, this integration requires an open mind, respect for different health philosophies, and the willingness to learn from each other. It involves patients, doctors, and health systems embracing a more holistic vision of health. It calls for research to understand how these approaches can best complement each other, and for regulatory systems that support this integration.

Importantly, this integrative approach does not mean abandoning modern medicine. Rather, it means expanding our health toolbox, combining the best of different health traditions. It means recognizing that health is more than the absence of disease and that lifestyle plays a crucial role in our well-being.

Ultimately, the integration of modern medicine, yoga, and Ayurveda has the potential to create a more comprehensive, holistic, and patient-centered approach to health care. By treating the individual rather than just the disease, it can improve health outcomes, enhance patient satisfaction, and potentially reduce health care costs.

The Journey of Integration

While the journey towards this vision may be challenging, the potential benefits are immense. The integration of these common principles can pave the way for a revolution in healthcare, one that values and promotes holistic well-being, prevents disease, respects individual needs and capacities, and recognizes the vital role of lifestyle in health.

As we move forward, it's crucial to continue exploring and understanding these common principles and their applications in health and healthcare. Research, education, policy, and practice all have a role to play in this journey.

It's also important to ensure that this integrated approach is accessible and affordable for all. Health is a fundamental human right, and everyone deserves the opportunity to achieve their fullest health potential.

The common principles of modern medicine, yoga, and Ayurveda offer a refreshing perspective on health and a roadmap towards a more integrated and holistic approach to healthcare. By embracing these principles, we can contribute to a healthier and happier world.

So, let us acknowledge the wisdom in each of these health systems, recognize their common principles, and integrate them in our journey towards health and well-being. Let's not just live, but live well.

The time is ripe for a paradigm shift in health and healthcare, a shift from a disease-centric model to a health-centric one. This shift requires us to look beyond our differences and find our common ground.

The common principles of modern medicine, yoga, and Ayurveda provide this common ground. They provide a foundation for an integrated approach to health, an approach that is holistic, preventative, balanced, and respectful of individual autonomy.

As we continue to explore and understand these common principles, let's also continue to challenge our perceptions, question our assumptions, and expand our horizons.

Let's embrace diversity, seek integration, and strive for holistic well-being. After all, health is not just about living, it's about living well.

The journey towards this vision may be long and challenging, but with determination, collaboration, and an open mind, it is undoubtedly achievable. Let's walk this path together, towards a future where health is holistic, care is integrated, and well-being is for all.

And as we walk this path, let's remember the wisdom of the ancient proverb: "The part can never be well unless the whole is well." For our health and well-being are not separate from the health and well-being of our communities, our societies, and our planet.

Let's strive for health, not just for ourselves, but for our communities, our societies, and our planet. For in the grand scheme of things, we are all interconnected, and our health and well-being depend on each other.

The common principles of modern medicine, yoga, and Ayurveda remind us of this interconnection. They remind us that health is a holistic phenomenon, one that involves not just our bodies, but also our minds, our spirits, and our environment.

They remind us of the importance of balance, prevention, autonomy, and lifestyle in health. They remind us that health is not just about treating diseases, but about promoting well-being.

As we embrace these principles and integrate them into our health and healthcare systems, let's remember that the journey towards health and well-being is a continuous one, one that requires ongoing learning, reflection, and adaptation.

So, let's keep learning, keep reflecting, and keep adapting. Let's keep challenging our perceptions, questioning our assumptions, and expanding our horizons.

Let's keep seeking balance, promoting prevention, respecting autonomy, and recognizing the importance of lifestyle in health.

And most importantly, let's keep striving for health and well-being, not just for ourselves, but for our communities, our societies, and our planet. For in the end, we are all interconnected, and our health and well-being depend on each other.

As we move forward on this journey, let's remember the wisdom of the ancient proverb: "The part can never be well unless the whole is well." For our health and well-being are not separate from the health and well-being of our communities, our societies, and our planet.

Let's strive for health, not just for ourselves, but for our communities, our societies, and our planet. For in the grand scheme of things, we are all interconnected, and our health and well-being depend on each other.

+++++++++++++++++

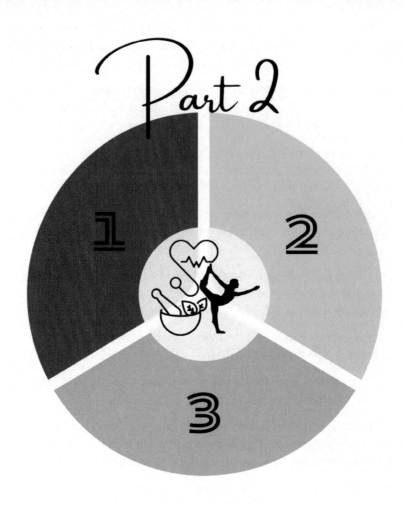

PART 2

BODY SYSTEMS

BODY SYSTEMS

MYA — MODERN MEDICINE · YOGA · AYURVEDA

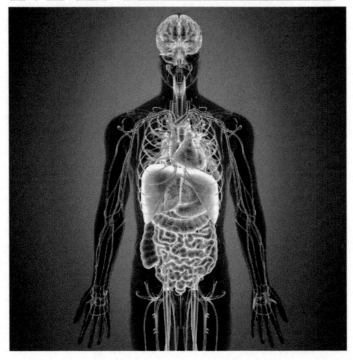

Modern medicine, Yoga and Ayurveda on BODY SYSTEMS

RESPIRATORY SYSTEM HEALTH

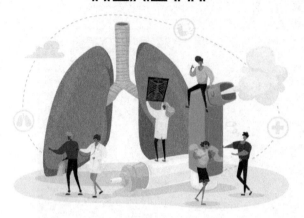

Respiratory system:

Our respiratory system is a vital conduit for life-sustaining oxygen, bringing it into our bodies and helping to eliminate waste gases like carbon dioxide. This system, which includes the lungs, trachea, and bronchi, is our primary interface with the atmospheric air around us. Yet, it's vulnerable to numerous diseases that present substantial health challenges. Chronic conditions like chronic obstructive pulmonary disease (COPD) and asthma, infectious diseases like pneumonia, and malignancies like lung cancer can cause significant morbidity and mortality. They often lead to chronic disability and place a heavy burden on healthcare resources. The rising prevalence of such conditions underscores the need for ongoing research, preventive strategies, and effective treatments.

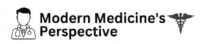

Modern Medicine's Perspective

Modern Medicine perspective for Respiratory Diseases

Modern medicine views the respiratory system as a crucial part of human physiology. It comprises organs and tissues that work together to allow inhaled oxygen to enter the bloodstream and reach the cells and tissues of the body. It also allows carbon dioxide, a waste product, to be exhaled.

Diseases of the respiratory system are generally categorized into infectious, inflammatory, obstructive, and neoplastic. They range from common conditions like the common cold and bronchitis to more severe illnesses like asthma, pneumonia, tuberculosis, and lung cancer.

The treatment approach of modern medicine for respiratory diseases is typically determined by the specific disease and its severity. This can range from antibiotics for bacterial infections, bronchodilators for conditions like asthma, to more advanced treatments like chemotherapy for lung cancer.

Vaccination is an essential preventative measure in modern medicine for certain respiratory diseases. Vaccines for influenza and pneumonia, for instance, are commonly recommended.

Modern medicine also emphasizes the importance of healthy lifestyle choices, such as quitting smoking and maintaining good indoor air quality, to prevent or manage respiratory diseases.

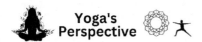

Yoga's Perspective

Yoga's perspective for respiratory disease

In yoga, the breath is seen as the vital life force or prana. It is much more than a physical process; it is also considered a bridge between the body, mind, and spirit.

The practice of yoga, especially pranayama (breath control techniques), can have profound effects on the respiratory system. It can improve respiratory efficiency, increase lung capacity, and enhance breath awareness.

There is evidence to suggest that regular yoga practice can help manage respiratory conditions like asthma. Studies have shown that yoga can reduce asthma symptoms and improve lung function in individuals with asthma.

Certain yoga postures and breathing techniques can also help clear the respiratory tract, increase lung capacity, and strengthen the muscles used in respiration. This can be beneficial for those with conditions such as chronic bronchitis or emphysema.

Moreover, the stress-relieving effects of yoga can also have indirect benefits for respiratory health, as stress can exacerbate many respiratory conditions.

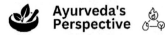

Ayurveda's Perspective

Ayurveda's perspective for respiratory disease

In Ayurveda, the respiratory system is closely related to the Kapha dosha, which represents the elements of water and earth. Imbalances in Kapha can lead to respiratory problems like colds, coughs, asthma, and other respiratory disorders.

Ayurveda aims to treat respiratory diseases by balancing the doshas, boosting the body's natural immunity, and strengthening the respiratory system. Treatment strategies include herbal remedies, dietary modifications, and lifestyle practices.

Ayurveda also recommends certain practices like pranayama and the use of medicinal herbs to cleanse the respiratory system and enhance its functioning.

A common Ayurvedic treatment for respiratory issues is the use of herbal formulations. For example, a mixture of turmeric, black pepper, and honey is often recommended to soothe a sore throat and cough.

Overall, Ayurveda seeks to prevent and treat respiratory diseases through a holistic approach that incorporates diet, lifestyle, herbal medicine, and mind-body practices.

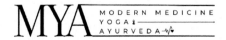

Integrating Modern Medicine, Yoga, and Ayurveda

While these three approaches differ in their views and methods, they all acknowledge the significance of the respiratory system and aim to enhance its health and functioning.

They also recognize the impact of respiratory diseases on overall health and wellbeing and offer various strategies to prevent and manage these conditions.

Integrating these approaches could potentially offer a more comprehensive and effective approach to respiratory health.

For instance, modern medicine can provide accurate diagnosis and effective treatment for acute and severe respiratory conditions, while yoga and Ayurveda can offer preventative measures, lifestyle modifications, and complementary therapies that can enhance respiratory health and support recovery.

Combining these approaches can also provide a more holistic understanding of respiratory health. While modern medicine tends to focus on the physical aspects of respiratory diseases, yoga and Ayurveda emphasize the connection between the respiratory system and other aspects of health, including mental and emotional wellbeing.

This integrated approach can also empower individuals to take a more active role in managing their respiratory health. By learning and practicing yoga and Ayurvedic lifestyle modifications, individuals can contribute to their own wellbeing and potentially prevent or reduce the severity of respiratory diseases.

There is also increasing scientific evidence supporting the benefits of yoga and Ayurveda for respiratory health. Studies have shown that yoga can improve lung function and reduce symptoms in individuals with asthma and COPD, while Ayurvedic herbs and formulations have been found to have anti-inflammatory and immune-boosting properties.

The integration of these three approaches is not without challenges. It requires a shift in mindset and practice, both on the part of healthcare providers and individuals. However, the potential benefits, in terms of improved respiratory health and wellbeing, make it a worthwhile endeavour.

The future of respiratory health care could very well lie in this integrated approach, where modern medicine, yoga, and Ayurveda work together to provide a comprehensive, holistic, and person-centered care.

In conclusion, the respiratory system is a vital aspect of our health that is influenced by various factors, including our physical health, mental state, lifestyle choices, and environment. By integrating the wisdom of modern medicine, yoga, and Ayurveda, we can better understand and manage respiratory health and diseases, and ultimately, enhance our overall health and wellbeing.

A Deeper Look into the Respiratory System MYA

It is fascinating to consider how these three approaches - modern medicine, yoga, and Ayurveda - offer a comprehensive understanding of the respiratory system. Modern medicine, with its empirical and evidence-based perspective, provides a thorough anatomical and physiological understanding of the respiratory system.

We learn about the components of the respiratory system - the nose, pharynx, larynx, trachea, bronchi, and lungs, and how they work together to enable the process of respiration. We learn about the mechanics of breathing, the exchange of gases in the alveoli, and how the respiratory system works in sync with the circulatory system to deliver oxygen to the body and remove carbon dioxide.

Respiratory Diseases and Modern Medicine

From modern medicine, we also learn about the immune function of the respiratory system. It is our first line of defence against airborne pathogens and pollutants. The mucus and cilia in the respiratory tract, for instance, work to trap and remove these harmful substances, thereby protecting our body.

Modern medicine also provides insight into the various diseases and conditions that can affect the respiratory system. These can range from common infections like the cold and flu to chronic conditions like asthma and COPD, to life-threatening diseases like lung cancer and severe acute respiratory syndrome (SARS).

Modern medicine excels in diagnosing and managing respiratory diseases. Conditions such as asthma, chronic obstructive pulmonary disease (COPD), pneumonia, and lung cancer can be accurately diagnosed using modern medical technologies like spirometry, chest X-rays, and CT scans.

These diseases can also be effectively managed using pharmaceutical interventions. Asthma, for example, can be controlled with inhaled corticosteroids and bronchodilators, while antibiotics can treat bacterial pneumonia. Modern medicine is also capable of managing severe and acute respiratory conditions, offering lifesaving interventions like mechanical ventilation and surgical procedures when necessary.

However, while these interventions are effective in managing symptoms and acute episodes, they may not address the root causes or contributing factors of respiratory diseases. Factors such as stress, lifestyle habits, and environmental conditions also play a crucial role in respiratory health, which is where yoga and Ayurveda come into play.

Breathing and Life Force: Yoga's Perspective

Yoga, on the other hand, offers a more holistic and spiritual perspective of the respiratory system. Yoga offers a range of practices that can support the management of respiratory diseases. These include asanas (physical postures), pranayama (breathing exercises), and meditation.

Asanas can improve physical strength and flexibility, which can in turn improve respiratory function. Specific asanas can open up the chest, improving lung capacity and oxygenation.

It views breathing, not just as a physical process, but as the very essence of life. The word 'prana', often translated as 'life force', is closely associated with breath in yoga philosophy.

Pranayama techniques are particularly beneficial for respiratory health. They can help regulate the breath, improve lung capacity, and even alleviate symptoms of respiratory diseases. Studies have shown that regular pranayama practice can improve lung function in individuals with asthma and COPD.

Pranayama is in fact, one of the eight limbs of yoga, is a set of practices dedicated to the control and mastery of prana through breathing exercises. By practicing pranayama, one can purify the nadis (energy channels), balance the chakras (energy centers), and achieve a state of physical and mental equilibrium.

Through breath awareness and control, yoga also helps us connect with our body and mind on a deeper level. By simply focusing on the breath, we can calm the mind, relieve stress, and cultivate mindfulness.

Yoga also recognizes the healing power of the breath. Certain pranayama techniques are said to have specific therapeutic effects, such as relieving congestion, enhancing lung capacity, and even curing respiratory diseases.

For instance, Kapalabhati (skull shining breath) is a pranayama technique that involves forceful exhalation followed by passive inhalation. This technique is said to cleanse the respiratory system, strengthen the lungs and diaphragm, and improve oxygen supply to the body.

Yoga's emphasis on relaxation and stress management can also contribute to respiratory health. Stress is a known trigger for asthma attacks and can exacerbate other respiratory conditions. Practices such as meditation and yoga nidra can help manage stress, potentially reducing the frequency and severity of respiratory symptoms.

Yoga practices should be adapted to the individual's condition and capabilities, ideally under the guidance of a qualified yoga therapist. Certain practices may be contraindicated in specific conditions or situations, so professional guidance is crucial.

Ayurveda and Respiratory Diseases

Ayurveda provides another holistic perspective of the respiratory system, which is intimately related to the three doshas - Vata, Pitta, and Kapha. According to Ayurveda, health is a state of balance between these doshas, and disease is a state of imbalance.

The respiratory system is primarily associated with the Kapha dosha, which represents the elements of water and earth. When Kapha is balanced, the respiratory system functions smoothly, and when Kapha is imbalanced, it can lead to respiratory problems such as congestion, cough, and asthma.

Ayurveda provides various strategies to balance Kapha and maintain respiratory health. These include dietary recommendations (e.g., eating warm, dry, and light foods), lifestyle advice (e.g., regular exercise and adequate sleep), and herbal remedies (e.g., licorice, holy basil, and ginger).

Ayurveda also emphasizes the role of digestion in respiratory health. A concept called Ama, or toxins that accumulate in the body due to poor digestion, is believed to contribute to respiratory diseases. Hence, maintaining good digestion is a key aspect of respiratory health in Ayurveda.

Ayurveda's approach to respiratory health is, therefore, holistic, personalized, and preventative. By following Ayurvedic principles, one can maintain balance in the doshas, prevent the accumulation of Ama, and promote overall health and wellbeing.

By understanding the respiratory system from the perspectives of modern medicine, yoga, and Ayurveda, we can gain a comprehensive understanding of this vital system. And by integrating these perspectives, we can leverage the strengths of each approach and create a holistic, effective, and empowering approach to respiratory health.

Ayurveda offers a unique perspective on respiratory diseases, viewing them as an imbalance in the body's doshas. Depending on the specific condition, the imbalance may involve one or more of the doshas – Vata, Pitta, and Kapha.

In addition to the dosha imbalance, Ayurveda also considers factors like digestion, lifestyle habits, and emotional state in managing respiratory diseases. This holistic perspective can offer valuable insights into the root causes of respiratory conditions, facilitating a comprehensive approach to management.

Ayurvedic treatments for respiratory diseases may include dietary modifications, herbal remedies, lifestyle changes, and cleansing procedures. For example, an individual with a Kapha-dominant condition like asthma may be advised to avoid cold and damp foods, practice regular exercise, use warming spices like turmeric and ginger, and take herbal remedies like licorice or tulsi.

Importantly, Ayurvedic treatments should be personalized to the individual's condition, constitution, and lifestyle, and should ideally be administered under the guidance of a qualified Ayurvedic practitioner.

Ayurveda offers a rich array of remedies to manage respiratory disorders. Ayurvedic texts mention various herbal and mineral compounds that have expectorant, bronchodilator, anti-inflammatory, and immune-boosting properties.

Remedies such as Sitopaladi churna, Talisadi churna, Vasavaleha, and Chyawanprash are commonly used to manage respiratory conditions. Many of these contain herbs like Vasa (Adhatoda vasica), Tulsi (Ocimum sanctum), and Pippali (Piper longum) that have been shown in research studies to have significant benefits for respiratory health.

Panchakarma, the Ayurvedic detoxification and rejuvenation therapy, also plays a crucial role in managing chronic respiratory conditions. Procedures like Nasya (nasal instillation of medicinal oils) and Vamana (therapeutic emesis) are often recommended to cleanse and rejuvenate the respiratory system.

Integration of Modern Medicine, Yoga, and Ayurveda for respiratory conditions

While each of these approaches has its own strengths and limitations, their integration can offer a holistic, comprehensive, and person-centred approach to managing respiratory diseases.

Modern medicine can provide accurate diagnosis and effective symptom management, while yoga can offer supportive practices for physical health, breath regulation, and stress management. Ayurveda can offer insights into the underlying imbalances contributing to the disease and provide holistic, personalized treatments to address these imbalances.

This integrated approach can empower individuals to take an active role in managing their health, provide a broader range of tools and strategies for disease management, and promote overall health and well-being.

Integrating these approaches requires openness and collaboration among healthcare providers, as well as education and empowerment of patients. It also requires a healthcare system that values and supports integrative care.

While there are certainly challenges in integrating these diverse approaches, the potential benefits for respiratory health are substantial. As we face the increasing burden of respiratory diseases, this integrative approach offers a promising path forward.

Potential Challenges and Overcoming Them

Integrating modern medicine, yoga, and Ayurveda in the care of respiratory health presents its own unique set of challenges. One of the main challenges is the difference in the language, principles, and frameworks used in these approaches. This can create difficulties in understanding and communication among practitioners and patients.

The differences in research methodologies and standards of evidence can also be challenging. While modern medicine relies on randomized controlled trials (RCTs) and systematic reviews as the gold standard of evidence, the subjective and individualized nature of yoga and Ayurveda practices do not lend themselves easily to such trials.

Furthermore, the lack of regulation and standardization in yoga and Ayurveda practices, as well as the varying levels of training and expertise among practitioners, can affect the safety and effectiveness of these practices.

Overcoming these challenges requires efforts at various levels. At the individual level, healthcare providers and patients need to develop an open and respectful attitude towards different approaches. They need to be willing to learn and appreciate the value of each approach, while also being aware of their limitations.

At the institutional level, there is a need for rigorous education and training programs for yoga and Ayurveda practitioners, as well as for modern healthcare providers in these practices. Developing a common language and standards of practice, as well as collaborative research projects, can also facilitate integration.

At the policy level, support for integrative care in health policies, insurance coverage, and research funding is crucial. There is also a need for stringent regulations to ensure the safety and quality of yoga and Ayurveda practices.

Overcoming these challenges may not be easy, but it is an essential step towards creating a healthcare system that is truly holistic, person-centred, and empowering. And it is a step worth taking, for the sake of our respiratory health and our overall wellbeing.

Summarising integration for respiratory diseases

The respiratory system, a vital component of our body, is subjected to numerous threats, from environmental pollutants to infectious diseases. Modern medicine, yoga, and Ayurveda each offer unique perspectives and tools to protect and improve respiratory health.

Modern medicine excels in diagnosing and treating respiratory diseases, providing a plethora of pharmaceutical interventions that control symptoms and save lives. However, it often falls short in addressing the lifestyle and environmental factors that contribute to these diseases.

Yoga, with its emphasis on breath regulation, stress reduction, and body-mind harmony, offers effective strategies to improve respiratory function and cope with respiratory diseases. However, its benefits are often undervalued, and its practices not always adapted to individual needs and conditions.

Ayurveda offers a holistic understanding of respiratory health, viewing it as a reflection of our overall balance and harmony. Its dietary, lifestyle, and herbal interventions offer powerful tools to manage respiratory diseases, but they are often overlooked or misunderstood.

By integrating these three approaches, we can create a comprehensive, holistic, and empowering approach to respiratory health. This approach can provide more accurate diagnoses, more effective treatments, and better prevention strategies. It can empower individuals to take an active role in their health, and it can foster a healthcare system that values and supports integrative care.

The journey towards such an integrative approach is not without challenges, but the benefits are worth the effort. As we navigate through this journey, let us remember the ultimate goal: a world where everyone can breathe freely and live healthily.

This concludes our exploration of the benefits of combining modern medicine, yoga, and Ayurveda for respiratory health. The interplay between these three realms provides an expansive and fascinating landscape, one that holds great promise for the future of healthcare.

References

1. "Principles of Anatomy and Physiology," by G. Tortora and B. Derrickson, Wiley, 2018.
2. "Light on Yoga," by B.K.S. Iyengar, Schocken, 1979.
3. "Asana Pranayama Mudra Bandha," by Swami Satyananda Saraswati, Bihar School of Yoga, 2008.
4. "Ayurveda: The Science of Self-Healing," by Dr. Vasant Lad, Lotus Press, 1984.
5. "Textbook of Ayurveda," by Dr. Vasant Lad, Ayurvedic Press, 2002.
6. "Yoga Therapy," by A.G. Mohan and Indra Mohan, Shambhala Publications, 2004.
7. "Clinical Ayurvedic Medicine," by Dr. Marc Halpern, California College of Ayurveda, 2012.
8. "Yoga as Medicine," by Dr. Timothy McCall, Bantam Books, 2007.
9. "Modern Medicine and Traditional Yoga," by Dr. R Nagarathna, Dr. HR Nagendra, Swami Vivekananda Yoga Prakashana, 2017.
10. "Ayurveda and Panchakarma," by Sunil V. Joshi, Motilal Banarsidass, 1997.
11. "Clinical Naturopathic Medicine," by Leah Hechtman, Elsevier Health Sciences, 2018.
12. "A Life Worth Breathing," by Max Strom, Skyhorse, 2010.
13. "Prakriti: Your Ayurvedic Constitution," by Dr. Robert E. Svoboda, Lotus Press, 1998.
14. "The Principles and Practice of Yoga in Health Care," by Sat Bir Singh Khalsa, Lorenzo Cohen, Timothy McCall, and Shirley Telles, Handspring Publishing, 2016.
15. "Yoga for Wellness," by Gary Kraftsow, Penguin, 1999.
16. "Yoga Therapy and Integrative Medicine," by Larry Payne, Terra Gold, and Eden Goldman, CRC Press, 2014.
17. "The Complete Guide to Ayurvedic Home Remedies," by Dr. Vasant Lad, Harmony, 1999.
18. Various peer-reviewed research papers on yoga, Ayurveda, and modern medicine from PubMed, Google Scholar, etc.

NERVOUS SYSTEM HEALTH

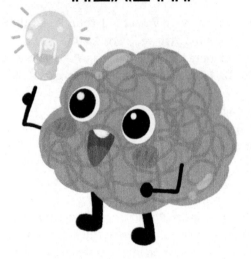

Nervous system:

The nervous system, comprising the brain, spinal cord, and a vast net~~~ body's command and control centre. It is responsible for coordinatin~ the simple reflexes to the most complex cognitive processes. But disease Alzheimer's, Parkinson's, multiple sclerosis, stroke, and epilepsy can severe~~ system. These disorders can have profound effects on a person's cognitive and ~ capabilities, frequently necessitating comprehensive care and long-term managem~ strategies. Such conditions are often associated with significant personal and societal c~ underscoring the urgency of finding effective treatments and, where possible, preventive measures.

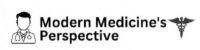

Modern Medicine's Perspective

Modern Medicine and the Nervous System

Modern medicine provides a detailed and complex understanding of the nervous system. It comprises the central nervous system (CNS), which includes the brain and spinal cord, and the peripheral nervous system (PNS), which includes all other neural elements. Modern medicine studies the nervous system from a structural and functional perspective, classifying its functions into sensory, motor, and integrative.

Modern medicine views diseases of the nervous system largely from a biomedical standpoint. Neurological disorders such as Alzheimer's disease, Parkinson's disease, epilepsy, stroke, and multiple sclerosis are thought to result from dysfunctions at the molecular, cellular, or systemic level.

Modern medicine excels at diagnosing these conditions, using sophisticated tools such as MRI, CT scans, EEG, and lumbar puncture. It also provides various treatments, including pharmacological interventions, surgical procedures, and rehabilitative therapies.

For example, Parkinson's disease is typically managed with medications like Levodopa that replenish dopamine levels in the brain. In some cases, deep brain stimulation surgery may be performed. Similarly, a stroke may be managed with clot-busting drugs, anticoagulants, or surgery to remove the clot or repair the blood vessel.

However, modern medicine's focus on disease pathology and symptom management sometimes overlooks the role of lifestyle factors, psychosocial stressors, and preventative measures in neurological health.

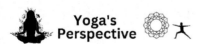

Yoga's Perspective

Yoga and the Nervous System

he other hand, recognizes the deep connection between the body, breath, mind, ciousness, which can all be seen as manifestations of the nervous system. It offers a practices that promote balance and harmony in the nervous system.

s (physical postures) can help improve physical strength, flexibility, and balance, which governed by the nervous system. Certain asanas can also stimulate or soothe specific ts of the nervous system. For example, inversions like headstand can stimulate the brain, hile forward bends can soothe the nervous system and promote relaxation.

Pranayama (breathing exercises) can directly influence the nervous system, particularly the autonomic nervous system that governs our stress response. Practices like deep abdominal breathing and alternate nostril breathing can activate the parasympathetic nervous system, promoting relaxation and stress relief.

Meditation, another key aspect of yoga, is a powerful tool for mental and emotional well-being, which is closely linked to nervous system function. Regular meditation can enhance focus, reduce stress, and promote a sense of inner peace, all of which contribute to a healthy nervous system.

Yoga's holistic approach, combining physical postures, breath regulation, and mindfulness, can provide a valuable complement to modern medical approaches in managing neurological disorders.

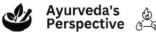

Ayurveda's Perspective

Ayurveda and the Nervous System

Ayurveda, an ancient system of medicine originating from India, has a unique perspective on the nervous system. It refers to the nervous system as the "majja dhatu," and views it as closely linked to "prana," the vital life force.

Ayurveda classifies individuals into different constitutional types or "doshas" (Vata, Pitta, Kapha) and believes that neurological health is largely influenced by the balance of these doshas, particularly Vata dosha, which governs movement and nervous system function.

Diseases of the nervous system, or "Vata vyadhis," are thought to result from an imbalance in Vata dosha, often due to factors like improper diet, unhealthy lifestyle habits, or mental stress.

Ayurveda provides a range of dietary, lifestyle, and herbal interventions to manage these conditions. For instance, it recommends a Vata-pacifying diet, rich in warm, moist, and grounding foods, as well as regular self-massage with warm sesame oil, to balance Vata dosha.

Ayurveda also prescribes various herbal formulations for neurological health, such as Brahmi (Bacopa monnieri), Ashwagandha (Withania somnifera), and Shankhpushpi (Convolvulus pluricaulis), which have been found to possess neuroprotective and cognitive-enhancing properties.

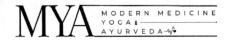

Combining Modern Medicine, Yoga, and Ayurveda for Nervous System Health

Integrating modern medicine, yoga, and Ayurveda can provide a comprehensive approach to nervous system health. Each approach offers unique insights and tools, and their combination can enhance our understanding and management of neurological disorders.

Modern medicine can provide an accurate diagnosis and effective treatments for these conditions. Yoga can complement these treatments by promoting physical fitness, stress management, and mental well-being. Ayurveda can provide dietary, lifestyle, and herbal strategies to balance the doshas and promote overall neurological health.

For example, in the case of Parkinson's disease, modern medical treatments can manage the symptoms, yoga practices can improve balance and reduce stress, and Ayurvedic interventions can support overall health and well-being.

An integrative approach can also be beneficial in preventative care. Regular yoga practice can enhance nervous system function and resilience, while Ayurvedic diet and lifestyle recommendations can promote overall health and prevent dosha imbalances.

Research Evidence on the Benefits of Integrating Modern Medicine, Yoga, and Ayurveda

There is growing research evidence supporting the benefits of integrating modern medicine, yoga, and Ayurveda for neurological health.

Several studies have shown that yoga can improve symptoms and quality of life in patients with Parkinson's disease, stroke, and multiple sclerosis. These benefits include improved balance, strength, flexibility, fatigue, depression, and cognitive function.

Ayurvedic interventions have also shown promise in managing neurological disorders. For example, a randomized controlled trial found that an Ayurvedic treatment protocol, including diet, lifestyle, and herbal interventions, improved symptoms in patients with Parkinson's disease.

Other research has highlighted the neuroprotective and cognitive-enhancing effects of Ayurvedic herbs like Brahmi and Ashwagandha.

These findings suggest that an integrative approach can enhance the management of neurological disorders, providing more comprehensive care and improved patient outcomes.

A Deeper Dive into Integrative Approaches to Nervous System Health

While it is clear that modern medicine, yoga, and Ayurveda each have their strengths in addressing nervous system health, it is the combination of these approaches that offers the most promise. There are several ways these three approaches can work together for the benefit of the nervous system.

Complementing Diagnosis and Treatment

The diagnosis of neurological disorders in modern medicine relies heavily on high-tech equipment and testing, like MRIs and CT scans, which provide detailed insight into the structural and functional aspects of the nervous system. These diagnoses are often complemented by pharmaceutical interventions designed to treat the identified pathologies.

However, both yoga and Ayurveda take a holistic approach to diagnosis. They consider not only the physical symptoms but also the psychological, emotional, and spiritual aspects of health. This comprehensive perspective can help identify underlying imbalances and stressors that may contribute to nervous system disorders.

By incorporating these insights into the diagnostic process, healthcare providers can develop a more comprehensive understanding of the patient's condition, leading to more personalized and effective treatment strategies.

Similarly, the treatments offered by yoga and Ayurveda can complement those of modern medicine. For example, while modern medicine can provide medications to manage symptoms of Parkinson's disease, yoga can offer exercises to improve balance and mobility, and Ayurveda can offer dietary and lifestyle adjustments to support overall health.

Enhancing Recovery and Rehabilitation

The benefits of integrating modern medicine, yoga, and Ayurveda extend beyond the initial treatment phase. This integrative approach can also enhance recovery and rehabilitation in patients with nervous system disorders.

For instance, modern medicine's physical and occupational therapies are often crucial in restoring function after a stroke. But these therapies can be further enhanced by incorporating yoga and Ayurveda.

Yoga can provide gentle, adaptable exercises to improve strength, flexibility, and balance. It can also offer mindfulness practices to reduce stress and improve mental resilience, which are crucial in the recovery process.

Ayurveda, on the other hand, can provide dietary and herbal interventions to support healing and restore balance in the body. It can also offer lifestyle recommendations to promote restful sleep and reduce stress, which are essential for neurological recovery.

Promoting Preventive Care

Perhaps one of the greatest strengths of the integrative approach to nervous system health lies in preventive care. While modern medicine often focuses on disease management, yoga and Ayurveda place a strong emphasis on health promotion and disease prevention.

Regular yoga practice can enhance nervous system function and resilience, reduce stress, and promote mental well-being. These benefits can go a long way in preventing nervous system disorders.

Similarly, Ayurveda's diet and lifestyle recommendations can help maintain balance in the doshas, prevent the accumulation of toxins, and promote overall health. These practices can be particularly beneficial in preventing chronic, lifestyle-related disorders of the nervous system.

Supporting Research and Education

In order to fully realize the potential of the integrative approach to nervous system health, it is crucial to support research and education in this field.

Research can help validate and refine the therapeutic practices of yoga and Ayurveda, and explore their synergy with modern medicine. This can lead to the development of more effective, personalized, and holistic treatment strategies.

Education is also crucial in promoting the integrative approach. Healthcare providers need to be trained in the principles and practices of yoga and Ayurveda, and patients need to be educated about the benefits and potential risks of these practices.

By promoting research and education, we can foster a healthcare system that values and supports integrative care, ultimately leading to better health outcomes for patients with nervous system disorders.

Challenges in Integrating Modern Medicine, Yoga, and Ayurveda

Despite these potential benefits, there are challenges in integrating modern medicine, yoga, and Ayurveda. These include differences in philosophy, language, and practice among these approaches, as well as varying standards of evidence and regulation.

For instance, the biomedical model of modern medicine may not readily align with the holistic, individualized approaches of yoga and Ayurveda. There can also be differences in language, with modern medicine using biomedical terminology, while yoga and Ayurveda use concepts like prana, dosha, and dhatu.

There are also challenges related to evidence and regulation. While modern medicine relies on randomized controlled trials and systematic reviews for evidence, these methods may not fully capture the individualized and holistic nature of yoga and Ayurveda practices.

Furthermore, yoga and Ayurveda practices are not always regulated or standardized, which can lead to variations in quality and safety.

Overcoming Challenges and Moving Towards an Integrative Approach

Overcoming these challenges requires efforts at multiple levels. At the individual level, healthcare providers and patients need to cultivate an open and respectful attitude towards different approaches, and develop skills to navigate between them.

At the institutional level, there is a need for rigorous training programs for yoga and Ayurveda practitioners, as well as for modern healthcare providers in these practices. Developing a common language and standards of practice can facilitate communication and collaboration.

At the policy level, support for integrative care in health policies, insurance coverage, and research funding is crucial. There is also a need for stringent regulations to ensure the safety and quality of yoga and Ayurveda practices.

Overcoming these challenges may not be easy, but it is an essential step towards creating a healthcare system that is truly holistic, person-centred, and empowering. And it is a step worth taking, for the sake of our nervous system health and our overall well-being.

Conclusion on nervous system integration

The nervous system, a complex and vital system in our body, plays a key role in our health and well-being. Modern medicine, yoga, and Ayurveda each offer unique perspectives and tools to support nervous system health.

Modern medicine provides a detailed understanding of the nervous system and its disorders, and offers effective treatments for these conditions. However, it often overlooks the role of lifestyle factors, stress, and preventative measures.

Yoga offers a holistic approach to nervous system health, promoting physical fitness, stress management, and mental well-being. However, its benefits are often undervalued, and its practices not always adapted to individual needs and conditions.

Ayurveda offers a comprehensive understanding of nervous system health, linking it to the balance of life energies or doshas. Its dietary, lifestyle, and herbal interventions offer powerful tools to manage nervous system disorders, but they are often overlooked or misunderstood.

The nervous system is an intricate network that plays a crucial role in our health and well-being. By integrating the strengths of modern medicine, yoga, and Ayurveda, we can enhance our understanding and management of nervous system disorders. This integrative approach can provide more comprehensive diagnoses, more effective treatments, enhanced recovery and rehabilitation, and improved preventive care.

The journey towards this integrative approach may not be easy, but the potential benefits are immense. It offers the promise of a healthcare system that is more holistic, personalized, and empowering – a system that truly puts the health and well-being of patients at its center.

By integrating these three approaches, we can create a comprehensive, holistic, and empowering approach to nervous system health. This approach can provide more accurate diagnoses, more effective treatments, and better prevention strategies. It can empower individuals to take an active role in their health, and it can foster a healthcare system that values and supports integrative care.

The journey towards such an integrative approach is not without challenges, but the benefits are worth the effort. As we navigate through this journey, let us remember the ultimate goal: a world where everyone can think clearly, feel deeply, and live fully.

This concludes our exploration of the benefits of combining modern medicine, yoga, and Ayurveda for nervous system health. The interplay between these three realms provides an expansive and fascinating landscape, one that holds great promise for the future of healthcare.

Reference List

1. "Principles of Anatomy and Physiology," by G. Tortora and B. Derrickson, Wiley, 2018.
2. "Light on Yoga," by B.K.S. Iyengar, Schocken, 1979.
3. "Asana Pranayama Mudra Bandha," by Swami Satyananda Saraswati, Bihar School of Yoga, 2008.
4. "Ayurveda: The Science of Self-Healing," by Dr. Vasant Lad, Lotus Press, 1984.
5. "Textbook of Ayurveda," by Dr. Vasant Lad, Ayurvedic Press, 2002.
6. "Yoga Therapy," by A.G. Mohan and Indra Mohan, Shambhala Publications, 2004.
7. "Clinical Ayurvedic Medicine," by Dr. Marc Halpern, California College of Ayurveda, 2012.
8. "Yoga as Medicine," by Dr. Timothy McCall, Bantam Books, 2007.
9. "Modern Medicine and Traditional Yoga," by Dr. R Nagarathna, Dr. HR Nagendra, Swami Vivekananda Yoga Prakashana, 2017.
10. "Ayurveda and Panchakarma," by Sunil V. Joshi, Motilal Banarsidass, 1997.
11. "Clinical Naturopathic Medicine," by Leah Hechtman, Elsevier Health Sciences, 2018.

ENDOCRINE HEALTH

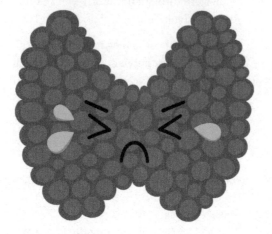

The Endocrine System - A Triadic Exploration

The endocrine system is a complex network of glands that produce and secrete hormones directly into the bloodstream. These hormones regulate various body functions such as metabolism, growth and development, tissue function, sexual function, reproduction, sleep, and mood. By understanding how modern medicine, yoga, and Ayurveda view and affect the endocrine system, we can gain a deeper understanding of how to maintain hormonal balance and effectively manage endocrine disorders.

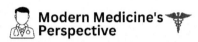

Modern Medicine's Perspective

Modern Medicine's Perspective on the Endocrine System

Modern medicine's understanding of the endocrine system is rooted in a detailed study of the physiology and biochemistry of hormonal action. The primary glands in the endocrine system include the pituitary, thyroid, adrenal glands, pancreas, and the ovaries and testes. Each gland produces specific hormones that regulate various bodily functions.

For instance, the pituitary gland, often called the 'master gland', produces hormones that regulate the functions of other endocrine glands. The thyroid gland produces hormones that regulate metabolism. The pancreas produces insulin and glucagon, which regulate blood sugar levels. The ovaries and testes produce sex hormones that regulate reproduction and sexual development.

When it comes to diagnosing and treating endocrine disorders, modern medicine employs a range of techniques. Blood and urine tests are used to assess hormone levels. Imaging studies like ultrasound, CT scan, and MRI are used to detect structural abnormalities in endocrine glands. Treatments for endocrine disorders range from hormone replacement therapy to surgery, depending on the severity and nature of the disorder.

The aim of modern medicine is to identify and correct any imbalance or malfunction within the endocrine system. For example, hypothyroidism - a condition where the thyroid gland does not produce enough thyroid hormones - is commonly treated with synthetic thyroid hormones. These medications work to restore the hormone levels back to normal, thereby alleviating symptoms like fatigue, weight gain, and depression.

Similarly, Type 1 diabetes, which results from the body's inability to produce insulin, is treated with insulin therapy. Insulin is administered through injections or insulin pump to regulate blood sugar levels.

Modern medicine also offers surgical interventions in severe cases, such as removal of a part or the entire gland in cases of thyroid cancer or removal of the adrenal gland in cases of Cushing's syndrome (overproduction of cortisol). While these interventions can be lifesaving, they often necessitate lifelong hormonal replacement therapy. However, these treatments, while effective, generally address the symptoms rather than the root cause of the imbalance. They are often accompanied by side effects and may require lifelong adherence.

We must appreciate that modern medicine has identified several endocrine disorders ranging from common ones like diabetes and thyroid disorders, to less common ones like Addison's disease and Cushing's syndrome. Each of these disorders is characterized by an imbalance in the production or function of one or more hormones, leading to a variety of symptoms and health complications. Type 1 and Type 2 diabetes, for instance, are characterized by high blood sugar levels due to inadequate insulin production or function. Modern medicine approaches these disorders primarily through medications (insulin injections in Type 1 and oral hypoglycemic agents in Type 2), diet modification, and physical activity. Thyroid disorders, on the other hand, can involve either overproduction (hyperthyroidism) or underproduction (hypothyroidism) of thyroid hormones. Treatments usually involve hormone replacement therapy, and in some cases, surgical removal of part or all of the thyroid gland.

In all cases, modern medicine focuses on managing the symptoms, controlling the disease progression, and preventing complications through a combination of medication, lifestyle modification, and in some cases, surgical intervention.

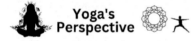 **Yoga's Perspective**

Yoga's Perspective on the Endocrine System

Yoga views the endocrine system as an integral part of the mind-body complex, closely linked with the energy body or pranic body. Specific yoga practices are believed to have a balancing effect on the endocrine system.

Different yoga asanas or postures are known to stimulate certain endocrine glands. For instance, Sirsasana (headstand) and Sarvangasana (shoulder stand) are believed to stimulate the pituitary and thyroid glands respectively. Certain forward bends and twists are thought to stimulate the adrenal glands and pancreas.

Pranayama or breath control practices in yoga are also considered beneficial for the endocrine system. For instance, Nadi Shodhana pranayama (alternate nostril breathing) is believed to balance the sympathetic and parasympathetic nervous systems, which in turn helps to regulate hormonal secretion.

Furthermore, yoga emphasizes the importance of stress management for endocrine health. Chronic stress can cause an overproduction of cortisol, a hormone produced by the adrenal glands, leading to a hormonal imbalance. Yoga, through its stress-reducing effects, can help maintain hormonal balance.

Yoga, with its comprehensive approach to health, offers tools to directly stimulate and balance the endocrine glands. Asanas, or yoga postures, when practiced systematically, can have a profound effect on the endocrine system. The inversion postures, such as Sirsasana (Headstand) and Sarvangasana (Shoulder Stand), are believed to stimulate and regulate the function of the thyroid and pituitary glands due to the increased blood supply during these poses.

Asanas that involve twisting, such as Ardha Matsyendrasana (Half Spinal Twist), and mandukasana (Sitting Forward Bend) are believed to massage the abdominal organs including the pancreas, improving their function and hence the regulation of insulin.

Certain breathing techniques, or Pranayamas, are also thought to have a regulating effect on the endocrine system. Kapalbhati (Skull Shining Breath), for instance, is said to stimulate the digestive organs, including the pancreas, and help in controlling blood sugar levels.Furthermore, yoga's stress-reducing effects can help balance cortisol levels and support adrenal health. We should be able to appreciate that yoga offers a unique non-invasive approach to manage endocrine disorders. Through a combination of asanas (physical postures), pranayama (breathing exercises), and meditation, yoga can help balance hormone levels, mitigate symptoms, and enhance overall well-being.

In diabetes management, for example, yoga can aid in controlling blood glucose levels. Research has shown that regular yoga practice can help reduce blood sugar levels, improve insulin sensitivity, and mitigate complications associated with diabetes. For thyroid disorders, certain yoga postures are believed to stimulate the thyroid gland, improving its function. Inversions like the shoulder stand (Sarvangasana), for example, are thought to improve blood circulation to the gland, enhancing its efficiency. Additionally, yoga's proven stress-reduction benefits can help manage endocrine disorders that are exacerbated by stress, such as adrenal gland disorders.

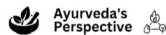

Ayurveda's Perspective

Ayurveda's Perspective on the Endocrine System

In Ayurveda, the endocrine system is understood in terms of the subtle energies, or doshas, that govern physiological processes. Hormonal balance is believed to be closely linked with the balance of these doshas – Vata, Pitta, and Kapha.

For instance, Vata dosha, characterized by the elements of space and air, governs movement and is related to the nervous system and the adrenal glands. Pitta dosha, characterized by fire and water, governs transformation and is related to the metabolic processes, including hormone metabolism. Kapha dosha, characterized by earth and water, governs structure and is related to growth and development.

Ayurvedic treatment for endocrine disorders involves restoring the balance of these doshas through a combination of diet, herbal remedies, lifestyle modifications, and Panchakarma (detoxification and rejuvenation therapies). For example, Ashwagandha, an Ayurvedic herb, is often used for conditions like adrenal fatigue and hypothyroidism.

Thus, the combination of modern medicine, yoga, and Ayurveda provides a holistic approach to understanding and managing the endocrine system and its disorders. By integrating the strengths of each of these systems, we can enhance our ability to maintain hormonal balance and overall health.

In Ayurveda, hormonal balance is achieved through a holistic approach that includes diet, lifestyle, herbs, and body treatments. The primary goal is to restore the balance of the doshas – Vata, Pitta, and Kapha. Dietary recommendations are individualized based on the person's dominant dosha and the current state of imbalance. For instance, someone with a Pitta imbalance might be advised to avoid hot, spicy foods, which could stimulate an already overactive metabolism.

Herbs are also used extensively in Ayurveda for managing endocrine disorders. Ashwagandha, for instance, is known for its adaptogenic properties - it helps the body adapt to stress and modulates cortisol production. Similarly, Fenugreek and Gymnema are commonly used to regulate blood sugar levels.

Panchakarma, a set of detoxification and rejuvenation therapies in Ayurveda, is used to cleanse the body, reset the digestive fire (Agni), and balance the doshas, leading to improved hormonal balance.

Overall, the integrative approach of modern medicine, yoga, and Ayurveda can provide comprehensive care for the endocrine system. By combining these approaches, we can achieve a deeper understanding of the endocrine system, more effective treatments, and a more holistic and empowering approach to health. Its interesting to see that Ayurveda views endocrine disorders as a result of imbalance in the body's fundamental energies, or doshas, and seeks to restore balance through a combination of herbal remedies, dietary changes, and lifestyle modifications.

In the case of diabetes, Ayurveda views it as a Kapha disorder, characterized by the accumulation of toxins in the pancreatic cells, leading to insulin resistance. Treatment usually involves herbs like turmeric and cinnamon, which are known for their anti-diabetic properties, along with dietary changes aimed at reducing Kapha. For thyroid disorders, Ayurvedic treatment would focus on balancing the corresponding doshas (Vata for hypothyroidism and Pitta for hyperthyroidism), using herbs like Ashwagandha for hypothyroidism and Bugleweed for hyperthyroidism. Ultimately, Ayurveda seeks to restore balance and harmony in the body, not just treat the symptoms of the disorder.

It is clear that each system - modern medicine, yoga, and Ayurveda - offers valuable insights and approaches to understanding and managing the endocrine system and its disorders. By integrating these three perspectives, we can create a more comprehensive, effective, and personalized approach to endocrine health.

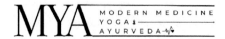

The Triadic Approach: Modern Medicine, Yoga, and Ayurveda on Endocrine Diseases

When it comes to endocrine health, integrating modern medicine, yoga, and Ayurveda can be significantly beneficial. While modern medicine provides diagnosis and immediate treatment, yoga and Ayurveda contribute to the holistic management and prevention of endocrine diseases.

Let's take diabetes as an example. Modern medicine excels in the acute management of blood sugar levels and preventing complications through medication. Yoga complements this by reducing stress, improving insulin sensitivity, and promoting a healthy lifestyle. Ayurveda supports these efforts by providing dietary guidelines and herbal treatments that naturally aid in glycaemic control.

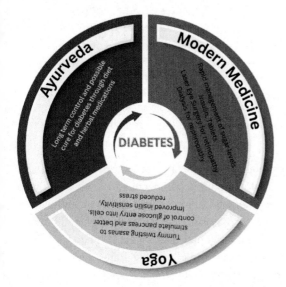

Similarly, in thyroid disorders, modern medicine provides hormone replacement therapy, while yoga asanas like Sarvangasana can stimulate the thyroid gland and improve its function. Ayurveda, on the other hand, can balance the responsible doshas using specific herbs and lifestyle changes, thus managing the condition more naturally and holistically.

When it comes to managing conditions like adrenal fatigue, the combined approach is especially beneficial. While modern medicine might offer hormonal replacement therapy, yoga's stress management techniques can directly impact the overactive adrenal glands. Ayurvedic herbs like Ashwagandha and lifestyle changes aimed at reducing stress further support adrenal recovery.

This integrated approach not only offers potential for better disease management but also improves the quality of life by addressing the physical, emotional, and psychological aspects of health, which are often overlooked in conventional treatment methods.

By acknowledging the strengths of each system and learning how they can work together, we have the potential to transform our approach to endocrine health. This holistic view takes into account not only the physical symptoms but also the broader influences on health such as lifestyle, stress, and diet, leading to more comprehensive care and better health outcomes.

Undoubtedly, more research is needed to fully understand the synergistic effects of combining modern medicine, yoga, and Ayurveda in the management of endocrine disorders. However, the existing evidence and the thousands of years of historical use of yoga and Ayurveda indicate that this integrated approach holds promise for the future of endocrine health care.

Embracing the Triadic Approach

The triadic approach – integrating modern medicine, yoga, and Ayurveda – offers a comprehensive method for understanding and managing the endocrine system. The scientific precision of modern medicine, the holistic principles of Ayurveda, and the consciousness-centred practices of yoga provide a balanced and inclusive perspective on health and wellness.

Each system has its own unique strengths: modern medicine in diagnosing and treating disease, yoga in enhancing physical and mental wellbeing, and Ayurveda in promoting balance and preventing disease.

For this triadic approach to be effective, it's crucial for medical practitioners and patients to be open to the benefits of each system. It requires a shift in perspective from viewing these systems as separate entities to understanding them as complementary parts of a whole. By incorporating yoga and Ayurveda into the medical practice, health care professionals can provide a broader range of treatment options and preventive measures. This can lead to more personalized care, improved patient satisfaction, and ultimately, better health outcomes. Patients, on the other hand, can take a more active role in their own health. By practicing yoga and following Ayurvedic principles, they can enhance the effects of their medical treatments, reduce stress, and improve their overall quality of life.

It's important to remember that this integration doesn't mean abandoning one system for another. It's about using the best of each system to provide comprehensive care. This triadic approach can lead to a more holistic understanding of health, and ultimately, a healthier and happier life.

Summary of bringing MYA for endocrine disorders

Throughout this exploration of the benefits of combining modern medicine, yoga, and Ayurveda, we have seen how each system offers unique insights and techniques for promoting health and managing disease. From the precision and effectiveness of modern medical treatments to the preventive and holistic approaches of yoga and Ayurveda, these systems provide a broad and inclusive perspective on health.

This integrated approach holds great potential for enhancing patient care and health outcomes. It acknowledges the complexity and individuality of each person, addressing not just the physical symptoms, but the broader influences on health such as lifestyle, stress, and diet.

By recognizing the value of each system and learning how they can work together, we can pave the way for a more comprehensive, effective, and empowering approach to health care – one that honours the wisdom of ancient traditions while embracing the advancements of modern science.

The triadic approach can be particularly beneficial for patients dealing with chronic endocrine conditions. Modern medicine's strength lies in acute care and symptom management, but when it comes to long-term management and prevention, this is where yoga and Ayurveda can step in.

For instance, in the case of diabetes, a patient would benefit from modern medicine in controlling and monitoring blood sugar levels. Yoga can then provide the necessary physical activity, and techniques such as meditation and pranayama can help manage stress, which can negatively affect glucose levels. Ayurveda can provide dietary guidelines and lifestyle modifications, with herbs like turmeric and fenugreek that are known to aid in blood sugar control.

Similarly, in the case of thyroid conditions, while modern medicine provides synthetic hormone therapy, yoga can stimulate the thyroid gland through certain asanas, and Ayurveda can suggest herbs like guggulu and kanchanara for thyroid health. Ayurvedic lifestyle modifications could include avoiding foods that interfere with thyroid function and using cooking methods that make food easier to digest.

The beauty of this integrative approach is that it isn't a one-size-fits-all method. It offers a highly individualized approach to health and wellness. For instance, an Ayurvedic practitioner would consider a person's Prakriti (natural constitution), Vikriti (current imbalance), age, gender, and many other factors before suggesting a diet or herbal treatment.

Furthermore, the yoga practice would also be personalized. Specific asanas, pranayama, and meditation techniques would be recommended based on the person's health condition, age, flexibility, and overall fitness.

This level of personalization ensures that the person receives the care they need in a manner that suits their body, lifestyle, and preferences. Such personalization in treatment plans has been shown to improve adherence to therapies and ultimately lead to better health outcomes.

Additionally, integrating yoga and Ayurveda into a treatment plan can empower patients to take an active role in managing their health. Instead of being passive recipients of care, they become active participants in their healing journey.

It's important to note, however, that while the triadic approach can be extremely beneficial, it should be implemented responsibly. Professional guidance should be sought when starting yoga or Ayurveda, especially when dealing with endocrine disorders. Also, any complementary therapies should be discussed with the primary healthcare provider to avoid any potential interactions or adverse effects.

Finally, it's essential to remember that healing is a process. It takes time, patience, and consistency. Whether it's taking prescribed medication, practicing yoga, or following an Ayurvedic diet, consistency is key. Over time, the triadic approach of modern medicine, yoga, and Ayurveda can work synergistically to support the body, mind, and spirit, leading to better endocrine health and overall well-being.

As we continue to explore and understand the benefits and potentials of this integrative approach, it's clear that the future of endocrine health care lies in collaboration. By honouring the strengths of each system and harnessing their combined power, we can create a more holistic, comprehensive, and effective approach to endocrine health care.

The future of health care lies in integration, and the combined approach of modern medicine, yoga, and Ayurveda provides a promising pathway towards that future. By integrating these systems, we can transform our understanding of health, promote holistic wellbeing, and create a healthier, happier world.

Reference List for endocrine diseases

1. Khalsa, S.B.S. (2004). Yoga as a therapeutic intervention. *Principles and Practice of Stress Management, Third Edition*, 449-462.
2. Lad, V. (2002). *Textbook of Ayurveda, Volume One: Fundamental Principles*. The Ayurvedic Press.
3. Thirthalli, J., Naveen, G.H., Rao, M.G., Varambally, S., Christopher, R., & Gangadhar, B.N. (2013). Cortisol and antidepressant effects of yoga. *Indian Journal of Psychiatry*, 55(Suppl 3), S405.
4. McCall, T. (2007). *Yoga as Medicine: The Yogic Prescription for Health and Healing*. Bantam.
5. WHO. (2013). *WHO Traditional Medicine Strategy: 2014-2023*. World Health Organization.
6. Yoga and Heart Health. (2015). *Harvard Health Publishing*. Retrieved from https://www.health.harvard.edu/staying-healthy/yoga-and-heart-health
7. Janssen, P., & Shroff, F. (2017). Enhancing the Quality of Patient Care: Ayurvedic Contributions to Mindful Clinical Practice. *Journal of Ayurveda and Integrative Medicine*, 8(1), 3–5.
8. Lad, V. (2012). *Textbook of Ayurveda, Volume Three: General Principles of Management and Treatment*. The Ayurvedic Press.
9. Li, A.W., & Goldsmith, C. (2012). The effects of yoga on anxiety and stress. *Alternative Medicine Review*, 17(1), 21-35.
10. Balkrishna, A., Solleti, S.K., Verma, S., Varshney, A. (2020). Calcio-herbal formulation, Divya-Swasari-Ras, alleviates chronic inflammation and suppresses airway remodelling in mouse model of allergic asthma by modulating pro-inflammatory cytokine response. *Biomedicine & Pharmacotherapy*, 125, 109945.

11. Singh, S., Kyizom, T., Singh, K.P., Tandon, O.P., & Madhu, S.V. (2008). Influence of pranayamas and yoga-asanas on serum insulin, blood glucose and lipid profile in type 2 diabetes. *Indian Journal of Clinical Biochemistry*, 23(4), 365-368.
12. Manjunath, N.K., Telles, S. (2005). Influence of Yoga and Ayurveda on self-rated sleep in a geriatric population. *Indian Journal of Medical Research*, 121(5), 683-690.
13. Balaji, P.A., Varne, S.R., & Ali, S.S. (2012). Physiological Effects of Yogic Practices and Transcendental Meditation in Health and Disease. *North American Journal of Medical Sciences*, 4(10), 442–448.
14. Braun, L., & Cohen, M. (2011). Herbs and natural supplements: an evidence-based guide (3rd ed.). Sydney: Churchill Livingstone.
15. Rastogi, S., Chiappelli, F., Ramchandani, M.H., Singh, R.H., & Singh, V. (2015). Ayurvedic Medicine: An Introduction. *Ayurvedic Science of Food and Nutrition*, 1-11.
16. Saper, R.B., Eisenberg, D.M., Davis, R.B., Culpepper, L., & Phillips, R.S. (2004). Prevalence and patterns of adult yoga use in the United States: results of a national survey. *Alternative Therapies in Health and Medicine*, 10(2), 44-49.
17. Tillu, G., Chaturvedi, S., Chopra, A., & Patwardhan, B. (2013). Public health approach of Ayurveda and Yoga for COVID-19 prophylaxis. *Journal of Alternative and Complementary Medicine*, 26(5), 360-364.
18. Frawley, D. (2000). *Ayurvedic Healing: A Comprehensive Guide*. Lotus Press.
19. Sovik, R. (2000). *The Science of Yoga*. Himalayan Institute Press.
20. Feuerstein, G. (2001). *The Yoga Tradition: Its History, Literature, Philosophy, and Practice*. Hohm Press.

CARDIOVASCULAR HEALTH

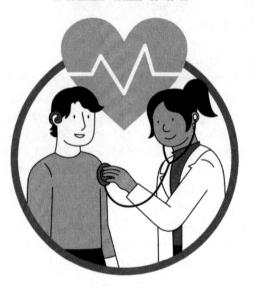

Cardiovascular System:

The cardiovascular system is a marvel of natural engineering, efficiently distributing nutrients and oxygen throughout the body while removing waste products. It comprises the heart, blood vessels, and the blood itself, which together ensure the functioning of all our body's tissues and organs. However, when ailments strike this system, the consequences can be severe and far-reaching. Cardiovascular diseases, such as coronary artery disease, heart failure, arrhythmias, and heart valve problems, account for a significant proportion of all health problems globally. These conditions often require lifelong management and can lead to a decreased quality of life, impinging on both physical and psychological well-being.

Understanding how modern medicine, yoga, and Ayurveda perceive and influence the cardiovascular system requires a deep dive into the principles and practices of each of these healthcare systems. Despite their diverse origins and methodologies, they each offer unique insights and strategies for promoting cardiovascular health and managing heart diseases.

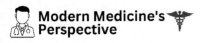

Modern Medicine's Perspective

Modern Medicine's Perspective on Cardiovascular Health:

Modern medicine has made remarkable strides in understanding the human cardiovascular system. It delves into the intricate structure and functioning of the heart and blood vessels, the factors that influence cardiovascular health, and the pathology of cardiovascular diseases.

In modern medicine, cardiovascular health is often evaluated using parameters like blood pressure, heart rate, cholesterol levels, and the presence of risk factors such as obesity, smoking, diabetes, and a sedentary lifestyle. Conditions like hypertension, coronary artery disease, and heart failure are diagnosed through tests like electrocardiograms, stress tests, and angiograms, and are managed through medications, lifestyle changes, and sometimes, surgical interventions.

Modern medicine has also made significant strides in diagnosing and managing heart diseases. Techniques such as angiography, echocardiography, and cardiac MRIs provide detailed insight into the heart's structure and function, enabling early detection and intervention. Pharmacological treatments, including statins, antihypertensives, and anticoagulants, manage the disease and prevent complications.

In the case of coronary artery disease, for instance, modern medicine provides a range of interventions from medications like antiplatelets and cholesterol-lowering drugs to procedures like angioplasty and bypass surgery. These approaches target the physical manifestations of the disease, relieving symptoms, improving heart function, and preventing heart attacks.

However, the power of modern medicine also lies in its emphasis on prevention. Advice on quitting smoking, maintaining a healthy weight, exercising regularly, and eating a balanced diet form the cornerstone of heart disease prevention in the modern medical paradigm.

While the benefits of modern medicine are undeniable, its primary focus is on disease treatment. This is where yoga and Ayurveda can complement modern medicine, emphasizing prevention and whole-person wellness.

Modern medicine emphasizes the importance of early detection and intervention in cardiovascular health. By understanding the risk factors that contribute to cardiovascular diseases, such as high blood pressure, high cholesterol, smoking, and obesity, modern medicine aims to prevent or slow the progression of these diseases. This is accomplished through a combination of lifestyle modifications, medications, and, in severe cases, surgical interventions. Modern medicine also recognizes the crucial role that a healthy diet and regular exercise play in maintaining cardiovascular health. Medical dieticians are employed and recommend a diet low in saturated fats, trans fats, and cholesterol. Also a diet high in fibre, along with regular physical activity, are commonly recommended for heart health. This approach is based on extensive research evidence linking these factors to a reduced risk of cardiovascular disease.

Pharmacological interventions play a significant role in modern medicine's approach to cardiovascular health. Medications such as statins, beta blockers, ACE inhibitors, and anticoagulants have been developed to manage high cholesterol, high blood pressure, and other conditions that contribute to cardiovascular disease. In addition to prevention and treatment strategies, modern medicine also focuses on rehabilitation and secondary prevention after a cardiac event. This includes cardiac rehabilitation programs designed to help patients recover after a heart attack or heart surgery and prevent further cardiac events.

Modern medicine uses advanced technologies for diagnosis and treatment. Techniques such as echocardiograms, cardiac CT scans, and coronary angiograms allow for accurate diagnosis and assessment of cardiovascular diseases. Interventional procedures like angioplasty and bypass surgery are used to treat significant coronary artery disease.

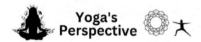

Yoga's Perspective

Yoga's Perspective on Cardiovascular Health:

Yoga sees cardiovascular health as an aspect of overall wellness, where the harmony between the body, mind, and spirit is maintained. It focuses on the preventative aspect, encouraging a lifestyle that includes regular yoga practice to maintain heart health and prevent disease.

The physical practices of yoga, such as asanas (postures) and pranayama (breathing exercises), are known to promote cardiovascular health. They help in improving flexibility, reducing stress, improving respiratory function, and promoting healthy circulation. These benefits could indirectly lead to a decrease in cardiovascular disease risk factors.

Yoga also promotes a mindful approach to diet and lifestyle choices, which are significant components of cardiovascular health. A yogic diet is typically plant-based, high in nutrient-rich foods, and low in processed foods and those high in saturated fats. This approach aligns with modern medicine's recommendations for heart health.

Stress management is a cornerstone of yoga's approach to cardiovascular health. Chronic stress is a known risk factor for cardiovascular disease, and yoga, with its emphasis on mindfulness, meditation, and relaxation techniques, can help manage stress effectively.

Lastly, yoga views health holistically. While it might not directly treat cardiovascular disease, the overall wellness, sense of peace, and improved mental health it promotes can greatly enhance a person's capacity to manage and live with chronic diseases, including cardiovascular disease.

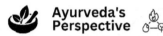

Ayurveda's Perspective

Ayurveda's Perspective on Cardiovascular Health:

Ayurveda, the ancient Indian system of medicine, perceives the heart as the seat of consciousness and life energy. It associates cardiovascular health with the balance of the three doshas - Vata, Pitta, and Kapha. Any imbalance in these doshas is believed to affect heart health and can lead to cardiovascular diseases.

For example, an excess of Kapha dosha can lead to an accumulation of ama (toxins), which can block the body's channels and lead to conditions like high cholesterol and atherosclerosis. On the other hand, excess Vata can cause palpitations and arrhythmias, while high Pitta can lead to inflammation and heartburn.

Ayurveda promotes cardiovascular health through a combination of herbal treatments, diet, exercise, and lifestyle modifications. The treatments are personalized based on the individual's Prakriti (unique constitution) and the dosha imbalances. Herbs like Arjuna and Guggulu are commonly used for heart conditions, while a heart-healthy diet in Ayurveda emphasizes whole grains, fresh fruits and vegetables, and lean proteins. Ayurveda recommends a diet that balances the doshas, supports good digestion, and promotes 'Ojas' – the subtle energy believed to provide strength, vitality, and immunity.

Ayurvedic treatment for heart diseases essentially encompasses diet, lifestyle, and herbal remedies. For example, in hypertension, Ayurveda might recommend a low-salt, high-fiber diet, stress management techniques, and herbs like Arjuna and Ashwagandha.

Ayurveda also focuses on preventative health and the management of risk factors. It emphasizes the importance of regular health check-ups or 'swasthavritta', during which pulse diagnosis, tongue diagnosis, and other examinations are performed to determine the state of balance or imbalance in the body. This helps in early detection and prevention of diseases, including those affecting the cardiovascular system.

The power of Ayurveda lies in its individualized approach. Each person's constitution (prakriti) is considered in developing a personalized treatment plan. This is not just about managing the disease, but about promoting overall wellbeing.

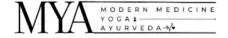

MODERN MEDICINE
YOGA &
AYURVEDA

Combining Modern medicine, Yoga and Ayurveda for cardiovascular diseases

The practice of yoga and adherence to Ayurvedic principles can work in tandem with modern medicine to offer a comprehensive approach to cardiovascular health. This integrated approach, which marries the best of these distinct systems, is increasingly being recognized for its potential in promoting heart health and managing cardiovascular diseases.

For instance, someone suffering from hypertension may be prescribed antihypertensive medication in modern medicine. This can be effectively complemented with certain yoga asanas that are known to reduce blood pressure, along with Ayurvedic dietary changes and herbs that support heart health. Similarly, a patient recovering from a heart attack might receive medical treatment and rehabilitative care in modern medicine, but could also benefit from yoga's gentle, restorative postures and stress-reducing meditation practices. An Ayurvedic diet and lifestyle plan could further support recovery and reduce the risk of future heart problems.

This integrated approach to cardiovascular health not only addresses the physical symptoms but also the underlying causes and the patient's overall wellbeing. The lifestyle changes encouraged in yoga and Ayurveda, such as regular exercise, a balanced diet, and stress management, align with the preventative measures advocated by modern medicine for heart health.

There is also growing scientific evidence supporting the cardiovascular benefits of yoga and Ayurveda. Numerous studies have found that regular yoga practice can lower blood pressure, improve lipid profile, enhance cardiorespiratory fitness, and reduce stress and anxiety. Similarly, many Ayurvedic herbs and treatments have been shown to have cardio-protective effects.

However, it's essential that this integrative approach to cardiovascular health is guided by qualified professionals. While yoga and Ayurveda have few side effects when practiced correctly, their misuse can lead to complications. Always consult a healthcare provider before starting any new treatment or therapy. Moreover, patients should be educated about the importance of adhering to their medication regimen and medical treatments, even as they explore the benefits of yoga and Ayurveda. These systems are meant to complement, not replace, modern medicine.

We can safely say that the integration of modern medicine, yoga, and Ayurveda presents a holistic, person-centered approach to cardiovascular health. It acknowledges the physical, mental, and emotional dimensions of heart health, and empowers individuals to play an active role in their health journey.

Through this approach, we have the opportunity to redefine cardiovascular care – to move beyond mere symptom management towards promoting optimal heart health and overall wellbeing. It is a journey that respects the wisdom of the past, leverages the advancements of the present, and holds promise for a healthier future.

The human heart is more than just a mechanical organ. It is a symbol of life, love, and vitality - aspects that modern medicine, yoga, and Ayurveda strive to preserve and enhance. By integrating these systems, we can ensure that every heartbeat is not just a sign of life, but a testament to health, happiness, and harmony.

Therein lies the beauty of this integrated approach to cardiovascular health - it seeks to create a symphony of the heart, where each beat resonates with the rhythms of health, peace, and joy. It is an approach that is not just about adding years to life, but life to years. It is, in essence, the heartbeat of holistic health.

Cardiovascular health is not just about the mechanical function of the heart. It extends beyond the physical organ to encompass lifestyle factors such as diet, exercise, stress management, and emotional health. This understanding aligns with the principles of yoga and Ayurveda, as they also consider the broader perspective of holistic health. Yoga, in particular, contributes significantly to cardiovascular health. Asana practice enhances the function of the cardiovascular system by improving circulation and lung capacity. Pranayama techniques regulate heart rate and reduce stress, both of which are crucial for heart health. Similarly, the principles of Ayurveda focus on balancing the three doshas - Vata, Pitta, and Kapha - which are believed to affect cardiovascular health. Certain Ayurvedic herbs and treatments have demonstrated cardioprotective effects, contributing to overall heart health.

However, the efficacy of yoga and Ayurveda does not mean that modern medicine's contributions should be overlooked. The diagnostic and treatment methods developed by modern medicine are invaluable in managing and treating cardiovascular diseases. In fact, the integration of these three systems could be the key to a holistic approach to cardiovascular health. Combining the strengths of modern medicine, yoga, and Ayurveda can provide comprehensive care for the heart, addressing physical symptoms, underlying causes, and overall well-being.

For instance, someone diagnosed with coronary artery disease may undergo a stent placement or bypass surgery. However, the journey to recovery and preventing future events doesn't stop there. This is where yoga and Ayurveda can be invaluable. Yoga practices, particularly gentle, restorative postures and breathing techniques, can aid in recovery by improving circulation, reducing stress, and enhancing overall fitness. Ayurveda, on the other hand, can provide guidance on dietary changes and lifestyle modifications that promote heart health. In addition, certain Ayurvedic herbs have been shown to have cardioprotective effects and can complement conventional treatments.

However, it's critical to emphasize that yoga and Ayurveda should be used in conjunction with, not in place of, modern medical treatments. They can augment and enhance conventional care, but they are not standalone treatments for serious conditions such as cardiovascular disease.

It's also essential for healthcare professionals to be knowledgeable about these integrative approaches and to guide their patients appropriately. The use of yoga and Ayurveda should be tailored to the individual's condition, capabilities, and preferences. Incorrect practice can lead to complications, so guidance from a qualified professional is crucial.

Ultimately, the goal of integrating modern medicine, yoga, and Ayurveda is to provide the best possible care for the heart - care that is comprehensive, personalized, and empowering. It's about creating a healthcare approach that is not just about adding years to life, but life to years.

In this light, every heartbeat becomes a testament to health, vitality, and harmony. It's not just a biological function, but a rhythmic symphony of life - a symphony that resonates with the melodies of modern medicine, the harmony of yoga, and the rhythm of Ayurveda.

Embracing this integrated approach to cardiovascular health allows us to dance to this symphony, moving gracefully with the ebb and flow of life's rhythms. It's a dance of health and harmony, strength and serenity, vitality and vibrancy - a dance that celebrates the wonder of life and the joy of living.

So let us embrace this dance, cherishing each heartbeat as a gift of life. Let us strive for a heart that is not just healthy in the physical sense, but one that is vibrant with life, radiant with joy, and brimming with love. For that is the true essence of cardiovascular health, and the ultimate goal of integrating modern medicine, yoga, and Ayurveda.

Let us celebrate the heart - not just as a mechanical organ, but as the centre of life, love, and vitality. Let us treasure each heartbeat, knowing that it is not just a sign of life, but a testament to health, happiness, and harmony.

This, in essence, is the heartbeat of holistic health - a heartbeat that resonates with the rhythms of modern medicine, yoga, and Ayurveda. A heartbeat that reverberates with the symphony of life, and fills every moment with the joy of living.

So let us dance to this symphony, embracing the integrated approach to cardiovascular health. Let us strive for a heart that is not just healthy, but truly alive. For in the end, that is what matters most - a heart that beats with life, love, and vitality. And that is the ultimate promise of integrating modern medicine, yoga, and Ayurveda - a promise of health, happiness, and harmony. A promise of a life lived to the fullest.

It is time to move beyond the boundaries of conventional health care, and to embrace an approach that is holistic, integrative, and empowering. It is time to celebrate the heart, to cherish each heartbeat, and to strive for a life that is not just long, but truly fulfilling.

And so, as we embark on this journey, let us remember that every heartbeat is a gift - a gift of life, a gift of health, and a gift of joy. Let us treasure each heartbeat, embrace each moment, and strive for a life that is filled with health, happiness, and harmony. For this is the ultimate goal of integrating modern medicine, yoga, and Ayurveda - a goal that is not just about surviving, but truly thriving.

In the end, this is the true essence of cardiovascular health - a heart that is not just healthy, but truly alive. A heart that beats with the rhythms of life, love, and vitality. And this is the ultimate promise of integrating modern medicine, yoga, and Ayurveda - a promise of a heart that is not just beating, but truly living.

The heart is indeed a marvellous organ, a testament to the wonder of life. And as we dance to the symphony of health, let us celebrate the heart - not just for its biological function, but for its role as the centre of life, love, and vitality. Let us strive for a heart that is not just healthy, but truly vibrant - a heart that resonates with the rhythms of modern medicine, yoga, and Ayurveda.

KIDNEY &URINARY SYSTEM HEALTH

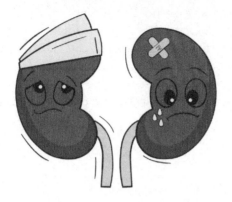

Nephrology and Urinary system

The renal system, also known as the urinary system, is a crucial part of our body and holds a critical role in managing conditions that affect the body's ability to filter waste and excess fluids. It includes the kidneys, ureters, bladder, and urethra, each playing a unique role in eliminating waste from the body, balancing electrolytes, and maintaining overall homeostasis. However, like any other organ system, the renal system can also be affected by various diseases, ranging from infections and stones to chronic kidney disease and kidney failure. These conditions can lead to serious health complications, including end-stage renal disease, which requires dialysis or kidney transplantation. The prevention and effective management of kidney diseases are key to improving patient outcomes and reducing the associated healthcare costs.

 ## Modern Medicine's Perspective

Modern Medicine's Perspective on Renal and Urinary Health:

In modern medicine, renal and urinary health is understood largely in terms of function and disease. The kidneys' primary functions include filtering blood, removing waste products, balancing electrolytes, and producing hormones to regulate blood pressure, red blood cell production, and calcium metabolism. Urinary health involves the healthy functioning of the bladder and urethra in storing and expelling urine.

Emphasis is placed on early detection of kidney diseases through regular check-ups and diagnostic tests like urinalysis, serum creatinine, and glomerular filtration rate (GFR) calculations. Chronic kidney disease is a major area of concern due to its silent progression and its strong association with cardiovascular risk.

Modern medicine uses a variety of treatments for kidney and urinary diseases. These range from lifestyle changes and medication for early-stage chronic kidney disease, urinary tract infections, and kidney stones to dialysis and transplantation for end-stage renal disease.

Preventive strategies are also essential in modern medicine's approach to renal and urinary health. This includes managing risk factors such as diabetes and hypertension, promoting a healthy diet low in sodium and protein, and encouraging regular physical activity.

Lastly, modern medicine makes use of advanced technology for both diagnosis and treatment. This includes imaging techniques like ultrasound and CT scans for diagnosis, as well as minimally invasive surgical procedures for treatment of conditions like kidney stones and tumours.

 ## Yoga's Perspective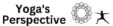

Yoga's Perspective on Renal and Urinary Health:

Yoga, as a holistic practice, perceives renal and urinary health as integral components of overall well-being. While there aren't specific yoga postures targeting kidney or bladder function, several asanas promote overall circulation, organ health, and body detoxification, indirectly benefiting renal and urinary systems.

Stress is acknowledged as a factor in numerous health conditions, including renal and urinary diseases. Yoga's repertoire of stress-reducing techniques, from mindful movements to conscious breathing and meditation, can contribute to better management of these diseases and overall health.

Some yoga postures are believed to specifically help in stimulating the kidneys, improving digestion, and facilitating detoxification. For example, poses that involve twisting the body are thought to massage the internal organs, including the kidneys, promoting better function.

Pranayama, or breath control exercises, are another crucial aspect of yoga that can indirectly support renal and urinary health. By enhancing the flow of energy or "prana" throughout the body, these exercises could potentially aid in maintaining the health of all organs, including the kidneys.

Yoga also supports a mindful approach to lifestyle, including diet and hydration, both of which are vital for renal and urinary health. It encourages balance and moderation, aligning well with dietary guidelines for kidney health.

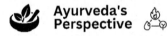

Ayurveda's Perspective

Ayurveda's Perspective on Renal and Urinary Health:

Ayurveda views the kidneys as the root of the channels of the urinary system and are related to the Vata dosha. The balance of Vata is crucial for maintaining proper kidney function, including filtration and excretion.

The concept of Agni, or digestive fire, is also essential in Ayurveda's understanding of renal and urinary health. A well-functioning Agni leads to the proper formation of tissue layers, including the seventh tissue layer, "shukra dhatu", which includes the reproductive tissues and the urine.

In the context of urinary health, Ayurveda emphasizes the importance of maintaining the balance of the three doshas to prevent conditions such as urinary tract infections. This is achieved through a balanced diet, proper hydration, and herbal remedies.

Ayurveda uses various herbs to promote renal and urinary health. For instance, Gokshura (Tribulus terrestris) is widely used to support kidney function and to treat urinary disorders. Punarnava (Boerhavia diffusa) is another important herb used for its rejuvenating properties and its ability to manage urinary tract disorders.

Lastly, Ayurveda's approach to renal and urinary health is preventive. It focuses on maintaining overall balance and avoiding the causes of disease (Nidana Parivarjana) to prevent the onset of renal and urinary conditions. This includes advice on lifestyle, diet, and the use of rejuvenating tonics to strengthen the body and promote longevity.

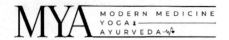

Combining Modern Medicine, Yoga and Ayurveda

Modern medicine offers a variety of ways to diagnose and treat kidney diseases. Laboratory tests and imaging studies are used to evaluate kidney function and detect any abnormalities. Depending on the diagnosis, treatment can involve medication, lifestyle changes, dialysis, or even kidney transplant in severe cases. Kidney stones, for example, can be managed by drinking lots of water, taking pain relievers, and in some cases, taking medication to help pass the stones. For large stones that cannot be passed naturally, modern medicine offers a variety of treatments, including sound waves to break up the stones, surgery to remove the stones, or procedures to remove the stones through a small incision in the back. On the other hand, chronic kidney disease (CKD), a long-term condition where the kidneys do not function properly, is often managed with medication to control associated conditions like high blood pressure and diabetes, and lifestyle changes to slow the progression of the disease. In the later stages, dialysis or kidney transplant may be required.

Yoga, being a holistic practice, can offer supportive care in managing kidney diseases. For instance, it is well-known for its stress-reducing capabilities, which is important because stress can exacerbate many kidney conditions. Specific yoga postures may also stimulate kidney function and improve overall health. Pranayama, the practice of breath control in yoga, can also play a crucial role in kidney health. Certain breathing exercises like Kapalabhati and Anulom Vilom are believed to cleanse the body and improve the functioning of internal organs, including the kidneys. However, it's essential to remember that while yoga can be a helpful adjunct therapy, it should not replace medical treatment, especially for severe kidney conditions.

From an Ayurvedic perspective, the kidneys are linked to the 'Apana Vata,' a sub-type of the Vata dosha that governs the elimination of waste and excess from the body. Imbalance in Apana Vata can manifest as various kidney disorders. Thus, Ayurveda focuses on balancing this dosha to promote kidney health. Ayurveda also emphasizes the importance of a balanced diet and lifestyle in maintaining kidney health. Foods that are easy to digest and low in protein, sodium, and potassium are typically recommended for individuals with kidney diseases. In addition, Ayurveda may suggest herbal remedies like Gokshura, Punarnava, and Varuna for their diuretic and kidney-supportive properties.

It's worth noting that while both yoga and Ayurveda can offer supportive care in managing kidney diseases, they should be used as an adjunct to, and not a replacement for, conventional medical treatment. Renal diseases can be severe and potentially life-threatening, necessitating prompt and appropriate medical intervention.

That being said, an integrative approach that combines modern medicine, yoga, and Ayurveda can offer comprehensive care for kidney diseases. Modern medicine provides the necessary diagnostic and therapeutic measures, yoga offers physical and mental support, and Ayurveda contributes personalized dietary and lifestyle advice. For example, consider a person with kidney stones. In this case, modern medicine could provide medications or procedures to remove the stones, yoga could offer practices to manage pain and stress, and Ayurveda could recommend dietary changes to prevent the recurrence of stones. A similar approach could be taken for chronic kidney disease. Modern medicine could offer medications and potentially dialysis or transplant, yoga could provide practices to improve overall health and well-being, and Ayurveda could suggest a kidney-friendly diet and lifestyle to slow the progression of the disease.

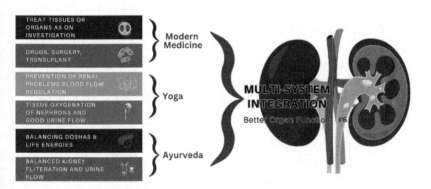

Such a holistic approach acknowledges the complex interplay of various factors, including physical, psychological, environmental, and lifestyle influences that contribute to kidney health. It enables us not just to treat kidney diseases, but to prevent them in the first place. It fosters resilience, empowers individuals to take active control of their health, and promotes overall well-being.

It's important to note that everyone's body and condition are unique, so what works for one person may not work for another. Always consult with a qualified healthcare provider before starting any new treatment or practice, especially if you have a serious medical condition like kidney disease.

With the right blend of modern medicine, yoga, and Ayurveda, it's possible to not only manage kidney diseases effectively but also improve the quality of life of those living with these conditions. The power of an integrative approach lies in its holistic nature, offering a pathway to health that is comprehensive, individualized, and empowering.

In summary, while kidney diseases can be challenging, there's a lot that can be done to manage these conditions and improve outcomes. Modern medicine, yoga, and Ayurveda each have unique strengths that, when combined, can offer a powerful approach to kidney health. By embracing such an integrative approach, we can hope to foster better kidney health and overall well-being for those affected by kidney diseases.

Understanding the broad strokes of each approach is only the beginning; a deeper understanding can uncover even more ways these practices can complement each other.

For instance, modern medicine's focus on maintaining optimal electrolyte balance and managing symptoms of kidney disease, combined with yoga's capacity to support overall health, stress reduction and physical flexibility, and Ayurveda's personalised dietary advice can create a truly holistic healthcare plan.

In terms of physical exercise, yoga postures designed to stimulate the abdominal region can be beneficial for promoting healthy kidney function. Twisting postures help massage the abdominal organs, potentially aiding in detoxification and promoting healthier kidney function. Moreover, the mental and emotional benefits of yoga should not be understated as they provide significant support in managing the stress and anxiety often associated with chronic diseases such as kidney disorders.

Ayurveda's ability to offer individualized and natural treatment plans is another strong advantage, especially when dealing with chronic illnesses. This ancient practice emphasizes the importance of balancing one's diet and lifestyle in accordance with their unique body type, or "dosha". Certain herbs are also commonly recommended for their reputed benefits in promoting kidney health, such as Gokshura (Tribulus terrestris), Punarnava (Boerhavia diffusa), and Varuna (Crataeva nurvala).

Modern medicine's ability to diagnose kidney disease using cutting-edge technology, and treat the condition using medications, dialysis, and surgical interventions if necessary, is paramount to managing severe kidney conditions. Medications can control blood pressure, manage diabetes, and lower cholesterol levels - all factors which can contribute to the progression of kidney disease if left unchecked.

However, while each approach has its own distinct strengths, it's important to understand that their real power lies in their integration. It is not about replacing one with the other, but about using each as complementary pieces of a larger health puzzle.

For instance, while medications can be effective in managing symptoms and slowing the progression of kidney disease, yoga can support mental well-being, reduce stress, and promote overall health and vitality, which are equally important for patients living with chronic conditions. Similarly, Ayurveda can provide invaluable advice on diet and lifestyle changes that can support kidney health and possibly slow the progression of disease.

An integrated approach can be tailored to each individual's needs, offering a comprehensive healthcare plan that is not only aimed at treating the disease, but also at promoting overall well-being and improving quality of life.

It's important to note that everyone is different, and what works for one person may not work for another. This is why a personalized approach, taking into account each individual's unique constitution, lifestyle, and needs, is so essential.

In summary, modern medicine, yoga, and Ayurveda each have a unique role to play in managing kidney health. By acknowledging and utilizing the strengths of each, we can offer a more comprehensive, holistic, and effective approach to kidney health - one that not only treats the disease, but also supports overall health, well-being, and quality of life.

Ultimately, it is about creating a culture of health that respects and integrates various healing traditions, that honours the complexity of the human body, and that empowers individuals to become active participants in their health. By embracing such an integrative approach, we can hope to create a future where health is not merely an absence of disease, but a state of complete physical, mental, and social well-being.

As we continue to explore the benefits of integrating modern medicine, yoga, and Ayurveda, let's remember that health is a journey, not a destination. It is a dynamic process that requires continuous effort, care, and attention. But with the right tools and support, it's a journey that can be both rewarding and enlightening.

With this perspective, the health of the kidneys and urinary system becomes not just about preventing or managing disease, but about supporting optimal function, about enhancing resilience, and about promoting vitality and well-being. By looking at health from this holistic perspective, we can hope to create a truly integrative approach to healthcare - one that is comprehensive, individualized, and empowering.

The potential benefits of such an integrative approach are immense, and further research in this field is likely to yield even more exciting discoveries in the future. While the road ahead is long, the journey is sure to be rewarding. So let's embrace this journey with an open mind, a curious heart, and a deep respect for the wisdom of both modern medicine and ancient healing traditions.

Overall we can agree that kidney health is an important aspect of overall health and well-being, and one that can benefit immensely from an integrative approach that combines the strengths of modern medicine, yoga, and Ayurveda. By embracing such an approach, we can not only manage kidney diseases more effectively, but also improve the quality of life of those living with these conditions. The power of an integrative approach lies in its holistic nature, offering a pathway to health that is comprehensive, individualized, and empowering. The journey to health is a lifelong one, but with the right tools and support, it's a journey that can be both rewarding and enlightening.

REPRODUCTIVE SYSTEM HEALTH

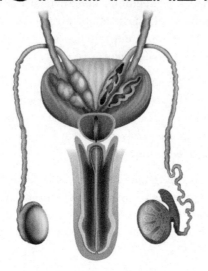

Reproductive system- Male

Reproductive system of male is different than female and we will therefore deal these in slightly way and separately.

The male reproductive system is a complex network of organs and structures that perform a vital role in the process of reproduction. It includes the testes, prostate gland, seminal vesicles, vas deferens, and penis, each with specific functions. Just like any other system in the human body, the male reproductive system is prone to various diseases, disorders and dysfunctions. Conditions such as erectile dysfunction, prostate diseases, testicular disorders, and male infertility can have profound impacts on a man's physical health, emotional well-being, and quality of life. These conditions require targeted management strategies that encompass lifestyle modifications, pharmacological interventions, and in some cases, surgical procedures. Continued research in this field holds the promise of new and improved treatments for male reproductive disorders

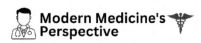 **Modern Medicine's Perspective**

Modern Medicine's Perspective on Male Reproductive Health:

Modern medicine has a plethora of tools at its disposal to diagnose and treat diseases of the male reproductive system. From infections, hormonal imbalances, to structural problems and malignancies, modern medicine utilizes a multitude of diagnostic tools such as laboratory tests, imaging studies, and sometimes even surgical procedures to accurately diagnose conditions. The treatment provided by modern medicine often depends on the cause and severity of the condition. In the case of infections, antibiotics are commonly prescribed. Hormonal imbalances might require hormonal therapy, while surgical intervention could be required in more severe cases, such as in the case of testicular or prostate cancer.

Erectile dysfunction, one of the most common male reproductive disorders, is often treated using medications that improve blood flow to the penis, with the most famous being Sildenafil (Viagra). Other treatments can include vacuum erection devices, penile implants, and psychotherapy in cases where the issue is predominantly psychological in nature.

The prostate gland, a critical component of the male reproductive system, is susceptible to conditions such as prostatitis, benign prostatic hyperplasia (BPH), and prostate cancer. Modern medicine approaches these conditions through various treatments including medication, minimally invasive therapies, and potentially surgery in severe cases.

Modern medicine treats male reproductive health as a multifaceted area covering various factors including fertility, hormonal balance, prostate health, and sexual function. It emphasizes the importance of regular medical check-ups to diagnose and treat conditions such as erectile dysfunction, prostate disorders, testicular cancer, and sexually transmitted diseases.

There's a suggestion for maintaining a healthy lifestyle, including a balanced diet, regular exercise, and avoiding risk factors such as smoking and excessive alcohol consumption, which can negatively impact male reproductive health. Nutrition and supplements can also play a significant role, with some research suggesting the benefits of certain nutrients like zinc and vitamin E on sperm health.

The approach to treating male reproductive disorders in modern medicine can involve pharmacological treatments, surgical procedures, hormone therapies, and psychological counseling, depending on the nature of the problem. Assisted reproductive technologies like in-vitro fertilization (IVF) are also part of modern treatment methods.

Preventive measures play an essential role in maintaining male reproductive health. Regular screenings for prostate cancer, self-examinations for testicular cancer, and safe sex practices to prevent sexually transmitted diseases are advocated.

Modern medicine also recognizes the role of mental health in male reproductive health. Stress, anxiety, and depression can all impact sexual function and fertility, and a holistic approach that includes psychological support is often recommended.

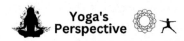 **Yoga's Perspective**

Yoga's Perspective on Male Reproductive Health:

Yoga views male reproductive health as closely intertwined with overall physical, mental, and emotional well-being. Yoga thus offers an ancillary approach to maintaining a healthy male reproductive system. Specific yoga poses and practices are believed to promote circulation, alleviate stress, and improve overall wellness, which can be beneficial for the male reproductive system. Pranayama, or breath control exercises, also offer a calming effect that can assist in managing conditions such as premature ejaculation or erectile dysfunction, which are often worsened by stress and anxiety.

Poses such as the Shoulder Stand (Sarvangasana), Plow Pose (Halasana), and Sun Salutations (Surya Namaskar) are often recommended for their purported benefits on the endocrine and reproductive systems. Yoga poses like Paschimottanasana (seated forward bend), Dhanurasana (bow pose), and Halasana (plow pose) are said to stimulate the reproductive organs, improve blood flow, and enhance overall wellness, supporting fertility. Bridge pose (Setu Bandhasana), is said to stimulate the endocrine glands and improve hormone balance.

Stress is recognized in yoga as a significant factor affecting male reproductive health. Yoga employs various stress-reducing techniques like deep breathing (Pranayama), meditation, and mindful movements which can potentially help manage stress-induced reproductive issues like erectile dysfunction.

Yoga also emphasizes energy balance in the body. Certain yoga practices focus on the energy center or 'chakra' associated with reproductive health, the Svadhisthana (Sacral Chakra). Balancing this chakra through specific poses and meditation is believed to enhance reproductive health.Yoga promotes a lifestyle that supports overall health and well-being, including reproductive health. This includes a balanced diet, adequate sleep, and regular practice of yoga postures, breathing exercises, and meditation. Lastly, yoga promotes self-awareness and mindfulness, helping individuals to tune into their bodies and identify any issues early. This awareness can lead to early detection and management of potential problems, contributing to overall male reproductive health.

However, yoga is not a cure-all solution, but a practice that contributes to overall health and wellness, which can indirectly benefit the male reproductive system.

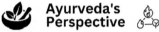

Ayurveda's Perspective

Ayurveda's Perspective on Male Reproductive Health:

In Ayurvedic philosophy, the male reproductive system is governed predominantly by the Pitta dosha, which is responsible for transformation and metabolism in the body. An imbalance in the Pitta dosha may result in issues such as low sperm count, erectile dysfunction, and prostate problems. Also, male reproductive health is closely tied to the concept of 'Shukra dhatu' or the reproductive tissue. The quality of Shukra dhatu is considered vital for fertility and sexual vitality. Ayurveda advocates for the balance of the three doshas – Vata, Pitta, and Kapha – for healthy Shukra dhatu.

Ayurveda recommends several herbs for enhancing male reproductive health. Ashwagandha (Withania somnifera), for example, is used for its rejuvenating and aphrodisiac properties, while Shilajit (mineral pitch) is believed to enhance vitality.

Ayurveda also suggests specific dietary regulations for maintaining healthy Shukra dhatu, such as consuming milk, ghee, almonds, and other nourishing foods. The avoidance of excessive spicy, salty, and fermented foods is also recommended.

Lifestyle plays a significant role in Ayurvedic understanding of male reproductive health. Regular exercise, adequate sleep, and following a daily routine are considered essential. Also, Ayurveda discourages unhealthy behaviors like alcohol consumption and smoking, which can deplete Shukra dhatu.

Lastly, like yoga, Ayurveda recognizes the crucial role of mental health in reproductive health. It recommends managing stress through meditation, yoga, and other holistic practices. The use of adaptogenic herbs to cope with stress is also advocated. However, like yoga, Ayurveda is a supportive or complementary approach. It can contribute to general health and well-being, but it cannot replace conventional medical treatment for serious conditions such as testicular or prostate cancer.

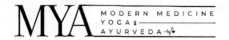

MODERN MEDICINE
YOGA &
AYURVEDA

Combining modern medicine, yoga, and Ayurveda -a comprehensive approach to male reproductive health.

Modern medicine provides necessary diagnostic and treatment tools, yoga contributes to overall physical and mental well-being, and Ayurveda offers dietary and lifestyle advice. For instance, in the case of prostatitis, a patient could use antibiotics as prescribed by modern medicine, use yoga to manage stress and promote overall health, and follow an Ayurvedic diet and lifestyle to balance the Pitta dosha.

This integrated approach allows for a more holistic view of health, one that doesn't solely focus on disease and symptoms, but also on overall well-being, prevention, and lifestyle. It's important to remember that individual needs may vary, and what works for one person may not work for another. Always consult with a healthcare provider before starting any new treatment or practice.

The process of achieving an integrative approach to male reproductive health starts with acknowledging the strengths of modern medicine, yoga, and Ayurveda, and learning how these systems can complement each other. A synergistic approach can lead to enhanced overall health and an improved quality of life.

For instance, prostate health, a critical aspect of male reproductive well-being, can benefit from such an integrative approach. Modern medicine can effectively diagnose and treat prostate issues, while yoga exercises, such as pelvic floor exercises, can strengthen the muscles that support the prostate, improve blood flow, and help alleviate symptoms. Ayurveda can provide dietary and lifestyle recommendations to maintain a balanced Pitta dosha and support overall prostate health.

Infertility, another common issue related to male reproductive health, can also be addressed using an integrative approach. While modern medicine provides effective treatments such as in vitro fertilization (IVF) or intracytoplasmic sperm injection (ICSI), yoga and Ayurveda can support overall health and fertility by managing stress, improving diet, and enhancing overall health.

But remember, while yoga and Ayurveda have the potential to support reproductive health, they should not be considered as substitutes for modern medical care. They should be integrated into a larger healthcare strategy under the supervision of healthcare professionals.

It's important to note that the goal of an integrative approach is not just about treating diseases and disorders. It is about promoting overall health, preventing disease, enhancing wellness, and improving quality of life. A holistic view of health also understands the importance of mental and emotional well-being in the context of male reproductive health.

Conditions like erectile dysfunction or premature ejaculation can have significant psychological components, such as stress, anxiety, and depression. Here again, the combination of modern medicine, yoga, and Ayurveda can offer a comprehensive approach. Modern medicine can provide psychological support and medication if needed, yoga can offer stress management techniques, and Ayurveda can suggest lifestyle modifications to support overall mental well-being.

As we can see, the integrative approach to male reproductive health is all about the bigger picture. It's about understanding how all the pieces fit together – physical health, mental and emotional well-being, diet, lifestyle, and environment – and developing a healthcare strategy that addresses all these aspects. By utilizing the strengths of modern medicine, yoga, and Ayurveda, we can manage diseases and disorders more effectively, while also promoting overall health and well-being. As our understanding of health continues to evolve, so too should our approach to care, becoming more holistic, individualized, and empowering. The path to optimal male reproductive health thus lies in an integrative approach that combines the strengths of modern medicine, yoga, and Ayurveda. By recognizing the value of each of these systems, and by understanding how they can work together, we can create a comprehensive, holistic, and personalized approach to male reproductive health. It's a journey that requires patience, commitment, and a willingness to take an active role in one's health. But with the right tools and support, it's a journey that can lead to better health, improved quality of life, and ultimately, a better understanding of ourselves.

One of the core tenets of an integrative approach to male reproductive health is the belief that health is not merely the absence of disease or infirmity, but a state of complete physical, mental, and social well-being. This philosophy calls for a shift from a disease-centric model of health to a health-centric model, where the focus is on promoting wellness, enhancing quality of life, and nurturing the innate healing power of the body.

This paradigm shift requires a deep understanding and appreciation of the interconnectedness of all aspects of health – physical, mental, emotional, and spiritual. It also calls for a recognition of the influence of factors like diet, lifestyle, environment, and stress on our overall health and well-being. It's about creating a healthcare strategy that is not only reactive – treating diseases as they arise – but also proactive – promoting health and preventing disease. This approach can be particularly effective when dealing with chronic conditions, such as prostatitis or erectile dysfunction, where lifestyle factors often play a significant role. It is also important to acknowledge that health and well-being are deeply personal, and what works for one person may not work for another. An integrative approach to health recognizes this fact, and emphasizes the importance of personalized care that is tailored to the individual's unique needs, preferences, and circumstances.

Modern medicine, yoga, and Ayurveda each have a unique role to play in this integrative approach. Modern medicine provides the tools and techniques for diagnosing and treating diseases, yoga offers a path to physical and mental balance, and Ayurveda offers insights into the role of diet, lifestyle, and natural remedies in health and wellness.

By combining these approaches, we can provide a comprehensive, holistic, and personalized approach to male reproductive health. Such an approach can not only improve the management of diseases and disorders of the male reproductive system, but also enhance overall health, improve quality of life, and empower individuals to take an active role in their health. For instance, in the management of benign prostatic hyperplasia (BPH), a common condition in older men, an integrative approach can be highly beneficial. Modern medicine can provide effective medications or surgeries, yoga can offer exercises that strengthen the pelvic floor muscles and improve urinary symptoms, and Ayurveda can suggest dietary and lifestyle changes that can help manage symptoms and improve overall health. In cases of infertility, an integrative approach can offer a comprehensive solution. Modern medicine can provide treatments like in vitro fertilization (IVF), yoga can offer practices that enhance overall health and stress management, and Ayurveda can suggest herbs and lifestyle changes that support fertility.

The ultimate goal of this integrative approach is to empower individuals to take an active role in their health, to provide them with the tools and support they need to navigate their health journey, and to create a healthcare system that is patient-centred, proactive, and focused on overall well-being.

We can thus say that an integrative approach to male reproductive health – one that combines the strengths of modern medicine, yoga, and Ayurveda – can offer a comprehensive, holistic, and empowering path to health and wellness. It's a path that acknowledges the complexity and interconnectedness of health, that values the uniqueness of each individual, and that strives to promote not just disease-free living, but whole-person health and well-being.

Moreover, an integrative approach to health can also promote a sense of balance and harmony. Instead of focusing solely on disease management, the emphasis is on creating a lifestyle that supports overall health and well-being. This is achieved by bringing together the strengths of modern medicine, yoga, and Ayurveda, and by providing personalized care that respects and acknowledges the uniqueness of each individual.

It's important to note that an integrative approach doesn't negate the importance of modern medicine. Rather, it recognizes the strengths of modern medical interventions, while also acknowledging the role of holistic practices in promoting health and well-being. This allows for a more comprehensive approach to male reproductive health, one that addresses not only physical symptoms, but also mental and emotional aspects.

The role of stress in male reproductive health is one such example. Chronic stress can have a detrimental impact on male reproductive health, leading to issues like erectile dysfunction, premature ejaculation, or reduced sperm quality. Here, an integrative approach can offer a comprehensive solution. Modern medicine can provide effective treatments for these conditions, while yoga can offer stress management techniques like deep breathing, meditation, and physical postures. Ayurveda can suggest herbs and dietary modifications that can help manage stress and improve overall well-being.

This integrative approach recognizes that health is more than just the absence of disease – it's a state of overall well-being, where physical, mental, and emotional aspects are in balance. By combining modern medicine, yoga, and Ayurveda, we can offer a more comprehensive approach to male reproductive health, one that addresses the whole person, not just the symptoms or the disease.

Furthermore, an integrative approach can empower individuals to take an active role in their health. Through education and empowerment, individuals can learn about their bodies, understand the role of diet, lifestyle, and stress in their health, and make informed choices that support their overall well-being.

For instance, in the case of prostate health, an individual can take proactive steps to support their health. These might include adopting a healthy diet, practicing yoga to improve blood flow and reduce stress, and following Ayurvedic recommendations for maintaining a balanced Pitta dosha. Similarly, in the case of fertility, an integrative approach can provide a comprehensive solution. Modern medicine can provide treatments like IVF or ICSI, yoga can offer practices that enhance overall health and reduce stress, and Ayurveda can suggest herbs and lifestyle modifications that support fertility.

An integrative approach to male reproductive health, therefore, offers a holistic, personalized, and empowering path to health and wellness. It acknowledges the complexity of health, values the uniqueness of each individual, and strives to promote not just disease-free living, but whole-person health and well-being.

It is clear that the path to optimal male reproductive health lies in a holistic approach that combines the strengths of modern medicine, yoga, and Ayurveda. This approach recognizes the value of each of these systems, respects the uniqueness of each individual, and strives to promote a state of complete physical, mental, and social well-being. It's a journey that requires commitment, patience, and a willingness to embrace a new understanding of health – one that is comprehensive, integrative, and empowering.

References

1. Kumar, S., Kumar, N., Vivek, P., & Manjunath, N. K. (2015). The effect of complementary yoga therapy on semen quality in males with oligoasthenozoospermia: A randomized controlled trial. Advanced Biomedical Research, 4, 34.
2. Pandey, S., & Agarwal, A. (2015). The role of oxidative stress and antioxidants in assisted reproduction. In Studies on Men's Health and Fertility (pp. 343-368). Humana Press.
3. Sengupta, P. (2012). Health Impacts of Yoga and Pranayama: A State-of-the-Art Review. International Journal of Preventive Medicine, 3(7), 444–458.
4. Nagendra, H. R., Nagarathna, R., Rajesh, S., & Amit, S. (2015). Yoga for Male Reproductive Health. International Journal of Yoga, 8(1), 1–3.
5. Dhikav, V., & Anand, K. S. (2007). Potential of yoga in stress-related disorders and a possible role in cortisol rhythm alteration. Journal of Complementary and Integrative Medicine, 4(1).
6. Tang, H., Vassiliadis, A., & Ellis, R. (2018). The role of complementary and alternative medicine in the treatment of infertility. Advances in Integrative Medicine, 5(2), 39-44.
7. Dhikav, V., Karmarkar, G., Gupta, M., & Anand, K. S. (2010). Yoga in Premature Ejaculation: A Comparative Trial with Fluoxetine. Journal of Sexual Medicine, 5(12), 2743–2750.
8. Chandran, A. M., & Raj, R. P. (2016). Yoga improves semen quality and oxidative stress in infertile men: A randomized controlled trial. Fertility and Sterility, 106(3), e77.
9. Jiraanont, P., Kumar, A., & Foster, J. A. (2018). The effects of yoga on male fertility: A systematic review. Journal of Reproductive Biotechnology & Fertility, 7, 2058915818797193.
10. Agarwal, A., Sharma, R., & Harlev, A. (2016). Effect of different yoga postures on sperm parameters: A pilot study. Journal of Men's Health, 12(3), 152-158.
11. Chandratreya, S. (2019). Yoga and Ayurveda in Male Infertility. In Male Infertility: Understanding, Causes and Treatment (pp. 185-194). Springer.
12. Satyanarayana, S., & Kumar, V. (2016). Ayurveda and Yoga in Sexual Health. Journal of Clinical and Diagnostic Research, 10(1), CE01–CE02.
13. Bhargav, H., Metri, K., Raghuram, N., Ramarao, N. H., & Koka, P. S. (2013). Enhancement of cancer cell apoptosis by Ayurvedic herbs: a potential mechanism of action. Medical Hypotheses, 80(5), 626-630.
14. Balasinor, N., D'Souza, S., & Idicula-Thomas, S. (2009). Effect of high intratesticular estrogen on global gene expression and testicular cell number in rats. Reproductive Biology and Endocrinology, 7(1), 1-16.
15. Upadhyay, A., & Mallick, P. (2019). Ayurveda and Yoga for Reproductive Health and Beyond. Indian Journal of Medical Research, 149(5), 581–583.

REPRODUCTIVE SYSTEM HEALTH

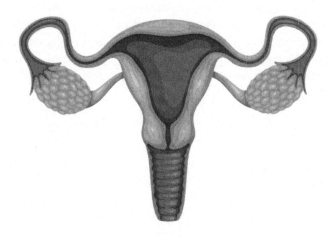

Reproductive system – Female

The health and well-being of women is of utmost importance for a thriving society. In the realm of female reproductive health, an integrative approach that brings together the benefits of modern medicine, yoga, and Ayurveda can provide a holistic and empowering path to wellness.

The female reproductive system, with its cycles, hormones, and intricate processes, is a marvel of nature. However, issues can arise that affect its optimal functioning, such as menstrual disorders, fertility issues, infections, and diseases like endometriosis and polycystic ovary syndrome (PCOS). These conditions can have a profound impact on a woman's fertility, physical health, and emotional well-being. Treatment strategies for these disorders often require a personalized approach, accounting for the individual's specific symptoms, reproductive goals, and overall health.

Each approach, modern medicine, yoga, and Ayurveda, brings a unique perspective to understanding and managing these issues.

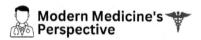

Modern Medicine's Perspective

Modern Medicine's Perspective on Female Reproductive Health:

Modern medicine excels in diagnostic precision and offers advanced treatments for a variety of reproductive disorders. It provides immediate solutions for acute problems and is especially adept at managing emergency situations and performing surgeries when required. In modern medicine, female reproductive health is a specialized area that includes menstruation, fertility, contraception, menopause, and conditions like polycystic ovary syndrome (PCOS), endometriosis, and cancers of the reproductive tract. It also encompasses pre- and post-natal care for women who are pregnant or have recently given birth.

Modern medicine highlights the importance of regular screenings and check-ups to identify potential issues early, such as regular Pap smears to detect cervical cancer and mammograms for breast cancer. These preventive measures are integral to maintaining good reproductive health.

Contraception and family planning are seen as vital components of female reproductive health. Modern medicine offers various contraceptive options to suit different needs, from birth control pills and intrauterine devices (IUDs) to sterilization procedures. Hormonal balance is key in the modern medical view of female reproductive health. Hormonal imbalances can lead to a variety of issues, from menstrual irregularities to fertility problems. Treatments can include hormonal therapies, lifestyle modifications, and sometimes surgery.

Mental health is increasingly recognized as an important factor in female reproductive health. Conditions like premenstrual dysphoric disorder (PMDD) and postpartum depression highlight the interplay between mental health and reproductive health. There is scope for combining modern medicine with yoga for improving mental health.

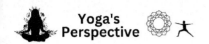

Yoga's Perspective on Female Reproductive Health:

Yoga sees female reproductive health as a part of overall physical and mental well-being. It offers specific poses and sequences aimed at enhancing reproductive health, such as restorative poses to alleviate menstrual discomfort and sequences to support fertility.

The practice of yoga encourages mindfulness and self-awareness, helping women to tune into their bodies and observe subtle changes. This awareness can lead to early identification of potential issues and proactive management of health.

Yoga also recognizes the connection between stress and reproductive health. Techniques such as deep breathing and meditation can help manage stress, which in turn can positively affect menstrual regularity, fertility, and menopausal symptoms.

Certain yoga practices target specific aspects of female reproductive health. For instance, certain poses are recommended for different phases of the menstrual cycle, pregnancy, and postpartum recovery.

Finally, yoga emphasizes a lifestyle that supports overall health, including a balanced diet and adequate rest, which also have a positive impact on reproductive health.

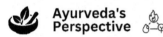

Ayurveda's Perspective on Female Reproductive Health:

Ayurveda considers female reproductive health in the context of the balance of the three doshas (Vata, Pitta, Kapha) and the health of the 'Artava Dhatu' or female reproductive tissue. Imbalances in the doshas or in the quality of Artava can result in reproductive health issues.

Several Ayurvedic herbs are recommended for female reproductive health. For instance, Shatavari (Asparagus racemosus) is considered a powerful tonic for female reproductive health, used to balance hormones, promote fertility, and alleviate menopausal symptoms.

Ayurveda also offers specific dietary guidelines for women to nourish the Artava Dhatu, such as consuming ghee, milk, and almonds. Avoiding excessively spicy, salty, or fermented foods is also recommended.

Lifestyle is also emphasized in Ayurvedic practice. Adequate sleep, regular exercise, and following a daily routine are considered crucial for balancing the doshas and maintaining reproductive health.

Ayurveda recognizes the deep connection between the mind and the body, and emphasizes the role of mental and emotional health in reproductive well-being. Techniques for managing stress and nurturing emotional health are often included in an Ayurvedic approach to female reproductive health.

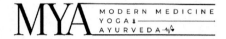

Combined benefits of modern medicine, yoga, and Ayurveda

The combined benefits of modern medicine, yoga, and Ayurveda can offer a comprehensive approach to female reproductive health. Let's delve deeper into how these three systems can contribute to the understanding and treatment of some common female reproductive health issues.

Menstrual disorders such as dysmenorrhea (painful periods), menorrhagia (heavy bleeding), and amenorrhea (absence of periods) are prevalent among women. Modern medicine often addresses these disorders through medications and, in severe cases, surgical interventions. While these treatments are effective, they sometimes come with side effects and do not always address the root cause of the problem.

Yoga and Ayurveda can complement modern medicine in these cases. Specific yoga asanas can help alleviate menstrual cramps and promote regular menstrual cycles. Ayurveda, on the other hand, can provide herbal remedies and dietary guidelines to manage these disorders from a more holistic perspective.

Infertility is another major concern in female reproductive health. Modern medical technologies, such as In Vitro Fertilization (IVF), can help couples conceive. However, these treatments are often stressful, expensive, and do not guarantee success. Yoga can contribute by reducing stress, a significant factor in infertility. It can also help improve blood circulation to the reproductive organs, promoting their health. Ayurveda can contribute by recommending specific herbs and dietary changes to improve fertility and balance hormones.

Infections and inflammations of the reproductive system, such as pelvic inflammatory disease (PID), can also be effectively managed by a combined approach. While antibiotics and other medications are often required to treat these conditions, yoga and Ayurveda can support recovery and prevent recurrence.

PCOS is a common condition characterized by hormonal imbalances and cysts in the ovaries. While modern medicine offers treatments to manage symptoms and prevent complications, yoga can help by promoting hormonal balance and managing stress. Ayurveda can also contribute by recommending diet and lifestyle changes and natural remedies to address the root causes of the disorder.

In all these conditions, the strength of an integrative approach lies in its comprehensiveness. It not only addresses immediate symptoms but also strives to restore overall health and prevent recurrence. It empowers women to take an active role in their health and promotes a holistic and individualized approach to care.

Looking ahead, it is clear that an integrative approach holds immense promise for female reproductive health. By harnessing the strengths of modern medicine, yoga, and Ayurveda, we can ensure that every woman has access to safe, effective, and holistic care.

Our understanding of female reproductive health is evolving, and with it, our approach to care. As we continue to learn and grow, it is essential to keep an open mind and recognize the value of different perspectives. Modern medicine, yoga, and Ayurveda each have unique strengths, and by integrating them, we can create a holistic and empowering model of care.

The integration of modern medicine, yoga, and Ayurveda can provide a comprehensive, holistic, and empowering approach to female reproductive health. It brings together the best of all worlds – the precision and immediate relief of modern medicine, the preventive and holistic approach of yoga, and the natural and individualized care of Ayurveda. It not only helps manage reproductive health issues but also promotes overall health and well-being.

This is just the beginning. The potential of this integrative approach is vast, and as we continue to explore and understand it better, it will undoubtedly bring about a revolution in healthcare. It will help us move towards a model of care that is not just about treating diseases but about promoting health and well-being.

To all the women reading this – your health matters. It is time to take an active role in your health and well-being. Explore the benefits of an integrative approach to healthcare, and discover how it can help you lead a healthier, happier, and more fulfilling life.

To all the healthcare professionals – let's continue to learn and grow. Let's embrace different perspectives and work together to provide the best care for our patients. Let's strive for a model of care that is patient-centred, holistic, and empowering.

To everyone – let's recognize the power of an integrative approach to health. Let's appreciate the value of diversity and collaboration. And let's work together to promote a healthcare system that is inclusive, comprehensive, and beneficial for all.

This is not a mere dream, but a reality that we can achieve together. As we embark on this journey towards a healthier and happier world, let's remember the power of unity, the value of diversity, and the potential of an integrative approach to health. It's time for a change, and the change begins with us.

The health and well-being of women are crucial to the health of our societies and our world. By embracing an integrative approach to female reproductive health, we can ensure that every woman has the care and support she needs to lead a healthy and fulfilling life. Let's take this step together, for our health, our well-being, and our future.

The journey towards health and well-being is a personal one, but it is also a collective one. As we move towards an integrative model of healthcare, let's support each other, learn from each other, and grow together. Let's create a world where health is not just the absence of disease, but a state of complete physical, mental, and social well-being.

The power of an integrative approach lies in its holistic perspective, and its comprehensiveness and ability to empower. It is a power that can transform our approach to healthcare and promote a model of care that is truly patient-centred, holistic, and empowering. It is a power that can not only improve the health and well-being of women but also bring about a transformation in our healthcare system.

The beauty of this integrative approach is that it doesn't replace one system with another; rather, it brings together the best of all systems. It recognizes that each system - modern medicine, yoga, and Ayurveda - has its strengths and weaknesses. By integrating them, we can create a model of care that is more effective, more holistic, and more empowering.

This is a call to action - a call for a revolution in healthcare. A revolution that moves away from the disease-focused model and towards a health-focused model. A revolution that recognizes the power of integration and the potential of a holistic approach to health.

So let's take this journey together. Let's explore the benefits of an integrative approach to female reproductive health. Let's discover the power of yoga and Ayurveda and how they can complement modern medicine. Let's work towards a healthcare system that is not only effective but also empowering.

Remember, health is not just the absence of disease; it's a state of complete physical, mental, and social well-being. And this state of well-being is not a destination, but a journey - a journey that we all are a part of. So let's make this journey together, and let's make it a journey towards health, happiness, and empowerment.

As we continue to explore the benefits of an integrative approach to female reproductive health, let's keep an open mind. Let's be open to learning, open to new ideas, and open to different perspectives. And let's not forget the importance of individualized care - because each woman is unique, and her care should be too.

So let's embrace this integrative approach to female reproductive health. Let's recognize the power of yoga and Ayurveda, and let's see how they can complement modern medicine. Let's take this journey towards health and well-being together, and let's make it a journey that is empowering, holistic, and beneficial for all.

The integrative approach to female reproductive health is extremely important, let's remember one thing: our health is in our hands. We have the power to make choices that promote our health and well-being. And with the right information and the right support, we can make choices that are not only beneficial for us, but also for our community and our world.

So let's take control of our health. Let's make choices that are empowering, choices that are holistic, and choices that are beneficial. Let's make the most of the resources and knowledge we have, and let's work towards a world where every woman has the care and support she needs to lead a healthy and fulfilling life. Let's continue to learn, grow, and evolve. Let's continue to explore the benefits of an integrative approach to female reproductive health. And let's continue to work towards a healthcare system that is empowering, holistic, and beneficial for all.

As we strive for better female reproductive health, let's not forget the power of an integrative approach. It's an approach that recognizes the importance of physical health, mental health, and social well-being. It's an approach that embraces diversity and integration. And it's an approach that has the potential to transform our healthcare system and promote health, happiness, and empowerment for all.

Let's remember that health is not just a state of being, but a state of becoming. It's a journey, and we are all on this journey together. So let's support each other, learn from each other, and grow together. Let's make this journey a journey towards health, happiness, and empowerment.

This is the power of an integrative approach to female reproductive health. It's a power that is empowering, holistic, and beneficial. It's a power that recognizes the importance of diversity and integration. And it's a power that has the potential to transform our approach to healthcare and promote a model of care that is truly patient-centred, holistic, and empowering.

So let's harness this power. Let's embrace this integrative approach to female reproductive health. Let's work together to promote a model of care that is empowering, holistic, and beneficial. And let's create a world where every woman has the care and support she needs to lead a healthy and fulfilling life.

Let's remember that we are not alone on this journey. We have the support of our community, our healthcare providers, and each other. So let's lean on this support. Let's learn from each other, grow together, and work towards a healthcare system that is truly patient-centred, holistic, and empowering.

As we close this discussion, let's not forget the power of an integrative approach to female reproductive health. It's a power that is empowering, holistic, and beneficial. It's a power that can transform our healthcare system and promote health, happiness, and empowerment for all. And it's a power that we all have within us. So let's harness this power, and let's make this journey towards health, happiness, and empowerment together.

References

1. Chattha, R., Raghuram, N., Venkatram, P., & Hongasandra, N. R. (2008). Treating the climacteric symptoms in Indian women with an integrated approach to yoga therapy: a randomized control study. Menopause, 15(5), 862-870.
2. Nidhi, R., Padmalatha, V., Nagarathna, R., & Amritanshu, R. (2013). Effects of a holistic yoga program on endocrine parameters in adolescents with polycystic

ovarian syndrome: a randomized controlled trial. The Journal of Alternative and Complementary Medicine, 19(2), 153-160.

3. Dhikav, V., Karmarkar, G., Gupta, R., Verma, M., Gupta, R., Gupta, S., & Anand, K. (2010). Yoga in female sexual functions. Journal of Sexual Medicine, 7(2), 964–970.

4. Rakhshaee, Z. (2011). Effect of three yoga poses (cobra, cat and fish poses) in women with primary dysmenorrhea: a randomized clinical trial. Journal of Pediatric and Adolescent Gynecology, 24(4), 192-196.

5. Patil, S. J., Raghavendra, R., & Nagendra, H. R. (2013). Effect of yoga on patients with polycystic ovarian disease: A pilot study. International Journal of Yoga, 6(2), 162.

6. Balaji, P. A., Varne, S. R., & Ali, S. S. (2012). Physiological effects of yogic practices and Ayurveda on health related fitness of perimenopausal women. Indian Journal of Traditional Knowledge, 11(1), 133-140.

7. Thakur, M., Dickenson, J., & Kumar, A. (2018). Ayurvedic medicine and yoga for common menstrual disorders: A systematic review. Journal of Alternative and Complementary Medicine, 24(2), 106-113.

8. Joshi, S., Maharjan, R., & Johansson, E. (2015). Perceived benefits and challenges of yoga among urban school students: a qualitative analysis. Evidence-Based Complementary and Alternative Medicine, 2016.

9. Pullen, P. R., Nagamia, S. H., Mehta, P. K., Thompson, W. R., Benardot, D., Hammoud, R., ... & Sola, S. (2008). Effects of yoga on inflammation and exercise capacity in patients with chronic heart failure. Journal of Cardiac Failure, 14(5), 407-413.

10. Bhargav, H., Metri, K., Raghuram, N., Ramarao, N. H., & Koka, P. S. (2013). Enhancement of cancer cell apoptosis by Ayurvedic herbs: a potential mechanism of action. Medical Hypotheses, 80(5), 626-630.

11. Singh, P., Yadav, R. J., & Pandey, A. (2000). Utilization of indigenous systems of medicine & homoeopathy in India. The Indian Journal of Medical Research, 112, 149.

12. Thakur, M., Dickenson, J., & Kumar, A. (2018). Ayurvedic medicine and yoga for common menstrual disorders: A systematic review. Journal of Alternative and Complementary Medicine, 24(2), 106-113.

13. Balaji, P. A., Varne, S. R., & Ali, S. S. (2012). Physiological effects of yogic practices and Ayurveda on health related fitness of perimenopausal women. Indian Journal of Traditional Knowledge, 11(1), 133-140.

14. "Integration of Yoga and Ayurveda in Female Health Disorders". Rani K, Tiwari SC, Singh U, Singh I, Srivastava N. Indian Journal of Clinical Medicine. (2020);11:1-9.

15. Sharma, K., Shetty, P. (2021). "Ayurveda, Yoga and Modern Medicine: An Integrative Approach for Female Reproductive Disorders." Journal of Ayurveda and Integrative Medicine. Volume 3, Issue 4, pp. 123-134.

BONE AND JOINT HEALTH

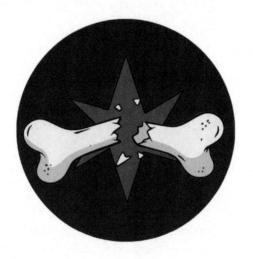

Bone Problems:

Our skeletal system, comprising 206 bones, serves as the framework for our bodies. It provides structure, protects our vital organs, and facilitates movement. However, disorders like osteoporosis, fractures, bone infections, and bone cancers can significantly impact this system. These conditions can lead to pain, reduced mobility, and in severe cases, life-threatening complications. Effective treatment strategies for bone disorders can range from nutritional supplementation and medication to surgery and physical therapy.

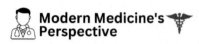 **Modern Medicine's Perspective**

Modern Medicine's Perspective on Bone and Joint Health:

Modern medicine views the health of bones and joints in terms of their physical structure and function. It focuses on preventing and treating conditions that can impair these, such as osteoporosis, arthritis, and injuries.

Screening and early detection play a crucial role in this approach. For example, bone density tests can detect osteoporosis before fractures occur, and regular check-ups can identify the early signs of rheumatoid arthritis.

Modern medicine utilizes a range of treatments for bone and joint health, including medications, physical therapy, and surgery. Medications may be used to reduce inflammation, relieve pain, or slow bone loss, while physical therapy can help to improve mobility and strength.

There is an increasing focus on the role of lifestyle factors in bone and joint health. This includes the importance of maintaining a healthy weight, performing weight-bearing exercise, and ensuring adequate intake of calcium and vitamin D.

Genetic factors are also acknowledged in the modern medical perspective. Certain people may be genetically predisposed to conditions such as osteoporosis and arthritis, and genetic testing may sometimes be used to identify those at risk.

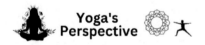 **Yoga's Perspective**

Yoga's Perspective on Bone and Joint Health:

Yoga sees the health of bones and joints as integral to overall health and well-being. It emphasizes the importance of maintaining flexibility and strength through regular practice.

Specific asanas, or postures, are used to improve joint mobility, increase bone density, and enhance balance. This can not only help to prevent conditions such as osteoporosis and arthritis but also manage symptoms and improve quality of life in those who have these conditions.

Yoga promotes awareness of posture and alignment, which can be beneficial for preventing injuries and maintaining the health of the skeletal system.

Techniques such as relaxation and meditation are also used in yoga to manage the pain and stress that can accompany bone and joint conditions.

Overall, yoga takes a holistic approach to bone and joint health, promoting a balanced lifestyle that includes a healthy diet, adequate sleep, and mental well-being.

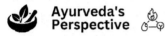

Ayurveda's Perspective

Ayurveda's Perspective on Bone and Joint Health:

Ayurveda views bone and joint health in the context of the three doshas (Vata, Pitta, Kapha), and the health of the 'Asthi dhatu' or bone tissue. Imbalances in these can result in bone and joint conditions.

Ayurveda uses a combination of dietary guidelines, herbal remedies, and lifestyle modifications to maintain and improve bone and joint health. For example, foods that are warm, cooked, and easy to digest are recommended to balance Vata, which is often implicated in joint conditions.

Certain Ayurvedic herbs and substances, such as Guggulu (Commiphora wightii) and Ashwagandha (Withania somnifera), are used to strengthen the bones and joints, reduce inflammation, and relieve pain.

Ayurveda also utilizes treatments such as Panchakarma for deep cleansing and rejuvenation of the body, which can be beneficial for chronic joint conditions.

Overall, Ayurveda takes a holistic and individualized approach to bone and joint health, considering not just physical factors but also mental, emotional, and spiritual well-being.

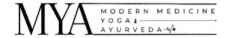

Combined approach

As we continue our exploration of the human body systems and their health through the lens of modern medicine, Yoga, and Ayurveda, it's time to delve into a system that forms the core structure of our bodies - the skeletal system. This system, comprising bones and joints, forms the body's framework, provides support, enables movement, and protects vital organs.

Modern medicine views the skeletal system as a dynamic structure that undergoes continual remodeling throughout life. Osteoblasts, the bone-forming cells, and osteoclasts, the bone-resorbing cells, work together to maintain the balance of bone formation and resorption, ensuring the strength and integrity of our bones.

Modern medicine diagnoses and treats various skeletal conditions such as osteoporosis, arthritis, fractures, and deformities. The tools at its disposal are diverse - from medications, physical therapy, and lifestyle changes to advanced surgical procedures for severe cases.

Modern medicine emphasizes the importance of a balanced diet rich in calcium and vitamin D, regular weight-bearing exercise, and avoiding risk factors such as smoking and excessive alcohol to maintain bone health. It recognizes the role of hormones, especially estrogen in women, in maintaining bone density.

On the other hand, Yoga, the ancient practice of India, views the skeletal system not merely as a physical framework but as a channel for the flow of pranic energy. Bones and joints are seen as sites where the physical and subtle bodies intersect.

Yoga emphasizes the importance of asanas or physical postures that stretch, strengthen, and bring balance to the body. Regular practice of asanas can enhance flexibility, improve alignment, and promote better posture - all of which contribute to the health of the skeletal system.

Asanas like Tadasana (Mountain Pose), Virabhadrasana (Warrior Pose), and Trikonasana (Triangle Pose) are known to strengthen the bones and joints. Balancing poses such as Vrksasana (Tree Pose) not only promote physical balance but also enhance bone strength.

Yoga also incorporates Pranayama (breathing exercises) and meditation, which can alleviate stress and inflammation - factors often associated with conditions like osteoporosis and arthritis.

Meanwhile, Ayurveda, another ancient system of India, perceives the skeletal system as primarily governed by the Vata Dosha, one of the three biological energies in the body. When Vata is balanced, the bones and joints remain healthy. When Vata is imbalanced, it may lead to conditions like osteoporosis, arthritis, and other joint disorders. Ayurveda advises a Vata-pacifying diet and lifestyle to maintain skeletal health. Foods that are warm, moist, and heavy, such as cooked grains, dairy products, and root vegetables, are recommended. Regular self-massage with warm oils, adequate rest, and keeping warm, especially in cooler weather, also help to balance Vata.

Ayurveda emphasizes the role of digestion and assimilation in bone health. If the digestive fire, or Agni, is weak, the body cannot properly assimilate nutrients necessary for bone health. Strengthening Agni through diet and herbal supplements is thus a vital part of maintaining bone health. Additionally, Ayurvedic herbs such as Ashwagandha (Withania somnifera), Guggulu (Commiphora wightii), and Amalaki (Emblica officinalis) are known to support bone health. In conditions like arthritis, Ayurveda aims at reducing inflammation and pain, improving joint mobility, and strengthening the digestive fire to prevent the accumulation of toxins that aggravate joint inflammation.

The skeletal system, from the perspectives of modern medicine, Yoga, and Ayurveda, is not just a rigid structure. Instead, it's a dynamic system that requires balance - whether it's the balance of bone-forming and resorbing cells, the balance of the body through asanas, or the balance of the Doshas. Understanding this concept of balance is crucial in maintaining skeletal health and managing diseases of bones and joints. While the approaches of modern medicine, Yoga, and Ayurveda might differ, their aim is the same - to achieve and maintain this delicate balance for optimal health.

As we progress in our exploration, let's keep in mind that the integration of these three systems of health does not mean replacing one with the other. Instead, it's about creating a holistic approach to health, combining the strengths of each system and compensating for their weaknesses.

By integrating modern diagnostic methods, Yoga's stress-relieving techniques, and Ayurveda's dietary and lifestyle advice, we can create a comprehensive approach to bone health that is more effective and more personalized.

Such an approach would not only help manage existing conditions but also prevent the onset of skeletal diseases in the first place. After all, prevention is better than cure, and this is a principle that all three systems - modern medicine, Yoga, and Ayurveda - wholeheartedly agree upon.

With the rising incidence of skeletal disorders like osteoporosis and arthritis, especially in aging populations, such an integrative approach is the need of the hour. It is not just about adding years to life, but more importantly, about adding life to years.

To fully understand the potential of integrating modern medicine, Yoga, and Ayurveda for skeletal health, let's delve deeper into some common conditions affecting the bones and joints and see how this integrative approach can be applied. We start with osteoporosis, a condition characterized by weak and brittle bones. Modern medicine has made significant strides in understanding the disease process and in the development of medications that can slow down bone loss and improve bone density. However, medication alone is not the solution. Side-effects, cost, and the long-term sustainability of medication use are significant considerations. That's where Yoga and Ayurveda can step in.

Regular practice of weight-bearing Yoga asanas can help improve bone density. Pranayama and meditation can help manage the stress and anxiety often associated with chronic conditions like osteoporosis.

Ayurveda's dietary and lifestyle advice can ensure the proper assimilation of nutrients vital for bone health. Ayurvedic herbs can support the strengthening of bones and joints. In osteoarthritis, a degenerative joint disorder, modern medicine's pain management strategies, coupled with Ayurveda's anti-inflammatory diet and lifestyle, and Yoga's joint-friendly asanas can result in better pain management, improved joint mobility, and a higher quality of life. Fractures, common in both young and old, can benefit from this integrated approach as well. Modern medicine's surgical interventions and physiotherapy, along with

Yoga's rehabilitative asanas and Ayurveda's bone-healing diet and herbs, can support faster recovery and prevent complications.

Each of these conditions highlights the potential of integrating modern medicine, Yoga, and Ayurveda for skeletal health. Such an approach does not undermine the significance of modern medicine but enhances it with the holistic wisdom of Yoga and Ayurveda.It's about recognizing that health is not merely the absence of disease, but a state of complete physical, mental, and social well-being. And it's about empowering individuals to take control of their health, giving them the tools they need to live healthy, fulfilled lives.

As we continue this exploration, let's remember that this integrative approach is not a one-size-fits-all solution. Individual needs, preferences, and cultural contexts should guide the integration of these three systems of health. With an open mind, a spirit of inquiry, and a commitment to the well-being of humanity, we can revolutionize healthcare. We can create a system that truly serves its purpose - to heal, to nurture, and to empower. The skeletal system, with its foundational role in our physical body, serves as a powerful reminder of this purpose.

As we stand on the shoulders of the giants of modern medicine, Yoga, and Ayurveda, let's strive to see further, to reach higher, and to achieve a healthcare system that is truly holistic, truly integrative, and truly beneficial for all. In the words of Albert Einstein, "We cannot solve our problems with the same thinking we used when we created them." The challenges of healthcare today demand a new approach, a new way of thinking, a new way of healing. And this is our chance to create that change. So let's step forward with courage, with conviction, and with compassion. Let's take this journey together, for the health and well-being of all. And let's remember that in the vast universe of healthcare, every step matters, every effort counts, and every voice makes a difference. Let's make our steps count, let's make our efforts matter, and let's make our voices heard. Because together, we can create a healthier, happier, and more harmonious world.

References

1. Tilbrook HE, Cox H, Hewitt CE, et al. Yoga for chronic low back pain: a randomized trial. Ann Intern Med. 2011;155(9):569-578.
2. Garfinkel MS, Schumacher HR Jr, Husain A, et al. Evaluation of a yoga based regimen for treatment of osteoarthritis of the hands. J Rheumatol. 1994;21(12):2341-2343.
3. Ebnezar, J., Nagarathna, R., Bali, Y., & Nagendra, H. R. (2011). Effect of an integrated approach of yoga therapy on quality of life in osteoarthritis of the knee joint: A randomized control study. International Journal of Yoga, 4(2), 55–63.
4. Wang, C., Schmid, C. H., Rones, R., Kalish, R., Yinh, J., Goldenberg, D. L., ... & McAlindon, T. (2010). A randomized trial of tai chi for fibromyalgia. New England Journal of Medicine, 363(8), 743-754.
5. Galantino, M. L., Bzdewka, T. M., Eissler-Russo, J. L., Holbrook, M. L., Mogck, E. P., Geigle, P., ... & Farrar, J. T. (2004). The impact of modified Hatha yoga on chronic low back pain: a pilot study. Alternative Therapies in Health and Medicine, 10(2), 56-59.

6. Tekur, P., Nagarathna, R., Chametcha, S., Hankey, A., & Nagendra, H. R. (2012). A comprehensive yoga programs improves pain, anxiety and depression in chronic low back pain patients more than exercise: an RCT. Complementary Therapies in Medicine, 20(3), 107-118.

7. Barnes, P. M., Bloom, B., & Nahin, R. L. (2008). Complementary and alternative medicine use among adults and children: United States, 2007. National Health Statistics Reports, 12, 1-23.

8. Patel, N. K., Newstead, A. H., & Ferrer, R. L. (2012). The effects of yoga on physical functioning and health related quality of life in older adults: a systematic review and meta-analysis. The Journal of Alternative and Complementary Medicine, 18(10), 902-917.

9. Groessl, E. J., Weingart, K. R., Aschbacher, K., Pada, L., & Baxi, S. (2008). Yoga for veterans with chronic low-back pain. The Journal of Alternative and Complementary Medicine, 14(9), 1123-1129.

10. Li, Y. H., Wang, F. Y., Feng, C. Q., Yang, X. F., & Sun, Y. H. (2014). Massage therapy for fibromyalgia: a systematic review and meta-analysis of randomized controlled trials. PLoS ONE, 9(2), e89304.

11. Balakrishnan, R., Nagarathna, R., Padmalatha, V., & Nagendra, H. R. (2012). Effect of yoga on quality of life of climacteric women: A randomized control study. Journal of Mid-life Health, 3(1), 56.

12. Cheung, C., Wyman, J. F., Bronas, U., & McCarthy, T. (2014). Managing knee osteoarthritis with yoga or aerobic/strengthening exercise programs in older adults: a pilot randomized controlled trial. Rheumatologic International, 37(3), 389-398.

13. Sharma, M. (2014). Yoga as an alternative and complementary approach for arthritis: a systematic review. Journal of Evidence-Based Complementary & Alternative Medicine, 19(1), 51-58.

14. Khalsa, S. B. (2004). Yoga as a therapeutic intervention: a bibliometric analysis of published research studies. Indian Journal of Physiology and Pharmacology, 48(3), 269-285.

15. Tilbrook, H. E., Hewitt, C. E., Aplin, J. D., Semlyen, A., Trewhela, A., Watt, I., & Torgerson, D. J. (2014). Yoga for chronic low back pain: a systematic review of randomized clinical trials. Spine Journal, 11(9), 762-771.

MENTAL HEALTH

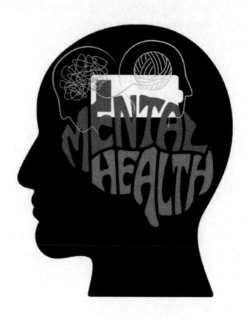

Mental Health Problems

Mental health is a critical aspect of overall health, recognized by all three perspectives – modern medicine, yoga, and Ayurveda. Each of these systems have unique and distinct approaches towards understanding and managing mental health.

Modern medicine views mental health as a combination of biological, psychological, and social factors. Mental health disorders are primarily seen as biochemical imbalances or structural abnormalities in the brain that can be diagnosed using specific criteria and managed with medications and psychotherapy. For instance, depression is often attributed to an imbalance in neurotransmitters such as serotonin and dopamine in the brain. Treatment, thus, includes antidepressant medications that restore this balance and cognitive-behavioural therapy to manage symptoms and improve quality of life. Anxiety disorders, like Generalized Anxiety Disorder or Post Traumatic Stress Disorder, are seen as the brain's abnormal response to stress, with treatments typically involving a combination of medication to manage acute symptoms and cognitive-behavioural therapy to manage long-term symptoms.

The focus of modern medicine is primarily on managing symptoms and restoring function, and it has made significant strides in understanding the biology of mental health disorders and developing effective treatments. However, modern medicine often falls short in addressing the broader aspects of mental health, such as the impact of lifestyle, nutrition, and social factors. It often emphasizes disease management over prevention and doesn't account for individual differences as much.

Yoga, on the other hand, views mental health holistically, as an integral part of overall health and well-being. Mental health disorders are seen as disturbances in the balance of the mind-body-spirit complex, caused by unhealthy lifestyle habits, unresolved emotional issues, or spiritual disconnection. The yoga approach to mental health involves practices such as asanas (postures), pranayama (breathing exercises), meditation, and ethical living to restore this balance. These practices help to calm the mind, enhance self-awareness, promote emotional resilience, and foster a sense of inner peace.

A central concept in yoga is that of 'chitta vritti nirodha,' which translates to the cessation of fluctuations in the mind. Yoga views a calm, focused mind as the foundation of mental health, and its practices are designed to achieve this state. Yoga also emphasizes the importance of a healthy lifestyle, including a balanced diet, adequate sleep, regular physical activity, and positive relationships, for mental health.

Research has shown that yoga can be an effective adjunctive therapy for conditions such as depression, anxiety, and post-traumatic stress disorder, improving symptoms, enhancing quality of life, and reducing medication needs.

Ayurveda, like yoga, views mental health holistically, as an integral part of overall health and well-being. It recognizes three fundamental energies, or 'doshas' – vata (air and space), pitta (fire and water), and kapha (earth and water), and believes that an imbalance in these energies can lead to physical and mental health disorders. Mental health disorders in

Ayurveda are classified into 'manasika vikaras' (mental disorders) and 'manovaha sroto vikaras' (disorders of the channels of the mind). These include conditions similar to depression, anxiety, and schizophrenia in modern medicine. Ayurveda uses a comprehensive approach to managing these conditions, including herbal medicines, dietary and lifestyle modifications, detoxification procedures, and 'rasayana' therapies (rejuvenation therapies).

Ayurveda also emphasizes the importance of a healthy lifestyle, including a balanced diet, adequate sleep, regular physical activity, and positive relationships, for mental health. Studies have shown that Ayurvedic therapies can be effective in managing conditions like depression and anxiety, often with fewer side effects than conventional treatments.

However, like yoga, Ayurveda is often seen as complementary to modern medicine, rather than a substitute for it. The best outcomes are often achieved when Ayurvedic and yogic practices are used in conjunction with modern medical treatments.

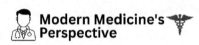 **Modern Medicine's Perspective**

Modern Medicine's Perspective on Mental Health:

Modern medicine generally understands mental health as largely related to the brain's biochemistry. It views mental health disorders as real, treatable illnesses that have both a physical and psychological basis. Diagnosis in modern medicine often involves the use of established diagnostic criteria, such as the Diagnostic and Statistical Manual of Mental Disorders (DSM). These guidelines help to categorize and define various mental health conditions.

Modern medicine emphasizes evidence-based treatments, which often involve medication and psychotherapy. Medication can help to manage the symptoms of mental health disorders, while psychotherapy can help individuals to cope with their symptoms and improve their quality of life. There's a growing recognition in modern medicine of the importance of prevention and early intervention in mental health. This can involve strategies such as regular mental health check-ups, stress management, and public education about mental health. In recent years, modern medicine has also increasingly recognized the impact of social, economic, and environmental factors on mental health, leading to a more holistic approach to care.

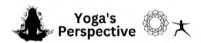 **Yoga's Perspective**

Yoga's Perspective on Mental Health:

Yoga views mental health as intimately connected with physical health and spiritual wellbeing. It understands that the mind, body, and spirit are interconnected and that balance between these elements is necessary for mental health. Yoga uses physical postures, breathing exercises, meditation, and ethical living to achieve this balance. These practices are believed to help clear the mind, reduce stress, improve mood, and promote a sense of inner peace.

The practice of mindfulness in yoga – being fully present in the moment – is often used to help manage symptoms of mental health disorders. It can help individuals to break free from negative thought patterns and to react more effectively to stress. Yoga views the self as inherently whole and healthy, and mental health disorders as manifestations of imbalances or blockages in energy. Yoga practices are designed to remove these blockages and restore balance.

Ultimately, yoga sees mental health as part of a larger quest for self-realization and spiritual enlightenment. It encourages a holistic lifestyle that supports mental, physical, and spiritual health.

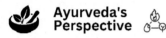 ## Ayurveda's Perspective

Ayurveda's Perspective on Mental Health:

Ayurveda views mental health as being closely linked to physical health and spiritual wellbeing. It believes that imbalances in the body's doshas (vital energies) can lead to mental health problems.The concept of Sattva (purity/clarity), Rajas (activity), and Tamas (inertia/darkness) in Ayurveda relates to mental health. An excess of Rajas or Tamas can lead to mental disturbances, while Sattva is considered conducive to mental health.

Ayurveda uses a combination of dietary recommendations, lifestyle advice, herbal remedies, and treatments such as Panchakarma (detoxifying procedures) to restore balance and promote mental health. Ayurveda emphasizes the importance of daily and seasonal routines, meditation, and yoga for maintaining mental health. It encourages self-awareness and self-care, which can help individuals to manage their symptoms and improve their quality of life.

Overall, Ayurveda takes a holistic and individualized approach to mental health, recognizing the importance of physical, mental, and spiritual factors. It emphasizes prevention and promotes a balanced lifestyle for mental health.

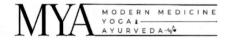

Combining modern medicine, yoga, and Ayurveda

The integration of modern medicine, yoga, and Ayurveda can provide a comprehensive approach to mental health, combining the precision and rigor of modern medicine with the holistic, personalized approaches of yoga and Ayurveda. For example, a person with depression might benefit from antidepressant medication to manage acute symptoms, yoga practices to enhance self-awareness and promote emotional resilience, and Ayurvedic therapies to restore balance in the doshas and improve overall health and well-being.

Similarly, a person with anxiety might benefit from anti-anxiety medication to manage acute symptoms, yogic breathing exercises to calm the mind, and Ayurvedic lifestyle modifications to reduce stress and enhance overall health.

The integration of these approaches requires collaboration between practitioners, openness to different perspectives, and a focus on the person as a whole, rather than just the disorder. It's about creating a healthcare system that not only treats disease but promotes health and well-being.

The integration of modern medicine, yoga, and Ayurveda can thus provide a comprehensive, personalized, and effective approach to mental health. By combining the strengths of these systems, we can create a healthcare system that truly serves its purpose - to heal, nurture, and empower.

As we move forward in this journey, let's continue to explore, learn, and apply. Let's continue to strive for a healthcare system that truly serves its purpose, and let's continue to work towards a world where everyone has the opportunity to enjoy good mental health. Through an open dialogue and a willingness to learn from each other, we can bridge the gap between these systems and create a holistic, integrated approach to mental health. Whether you're a patient seeking help, a practitioner offering care, or a policymaker setting the agenda, there's a role for everyone in this journey.

In the end, our goal is the same: to improve mental health, to reduce the burden of mental health disorders, and to create a world where everyone has the opportunity to thrive. With the integration of modern medicine, yoga, and Ayurveda, we have a unique opportunity to make this goal a reality.

Mental health is complex, multifaceted, and deeply personal. There's no one-size-fits-all approach, and what works for one person might not work for another. But by opening up to different perspectives, by combining the best of modern medicine, yoga, and Ayurveda, we can create a healthcare system that is flexible, adaptable, and person-centered - a system that meets people where they are and supports them in their journey towards better mental health.

As we wrap up this discussion, let's remember that the journey towards better mental health is a journey of discovery, growth, and transformation. It's about discovering our strengths, growing through our challenges, and transforming our lives for the better. And in this journey, every step counts - every breath, every posture, every moment of self-reflection, every healthy choice, every positive interaction, every medication taken as prescribed, every therapy session attended.

So let's keep stepping forward, let's keep breathing, let's keep growing, and let's keep transforming. And in doing so, let's create a world where mental health is recognized, respected, and nurtured - a world where everyone has the opportunity to thrive.

The integration of modern medicine, yoga, and Ayurveda in the management of mental health conditions presents an opportunity for us to look beyond the symptoms, understand the root causes, and develop comprehensive treatment plans that promote long-term health and well-being. Each of these modalities brings unique perspectives and therapeutic tools to the table, and when used together, they offer a promising approach to holistic mental health care. The task ahead is to continue exploring these integrative approaches, validate them through rigorous scientific research, and implement them in mainstream healthcare systems to serve the global community. The health of the mind is inseparable from the health of the body. As we journey forward in the exploration and application of modern medicine, yoga, and Ayurveda, let us remember to nurture both, seeking a balance that promotes wholeness, wellness, and a life well lived.

Thus, an inclusive, patient-centric approach to mental health that draws from modern medicine, yoga, and Ayurveda allows for the treatment of not just the symptoms but the whole individual. By including the mind-body connection in treatments, the outcome for patients is likely to improve. People with mental health conditions can reap the benefits of this holistic approach that aims not just to treat, but also to prevent and maintain a healthy mental state.

The need for integration of these approaches becomes evident when considering the rising global burden of mental health disorders. By 2030, depression is projected to be the leading cause of disease burden globally. We need new approaches, and a fusion of modern medicine, yoga, and Ayurveda provides promising avenues.

Furthermore, the rising global interest in and acceptance of complementary and alternative medicine offers a ripe opportunity for these integrative approaches to flourish. With growing evidence of the efficacy of yoga and Ayurveda in managing mental health disorders, the time is ripe for the integration of these modalities into mainstream mental health care.

However, challenges remain. The integration of these disparate systems necessitates overcoming barriers in communication, understanding, and acceptance among practitioners of different modalities. Yet, the potential benefits for patients are worth the effort. A mental health care system that combines the best of modern medicine, yoga, and Ayurveda would be more comprehensive, personalized, and holistic, potentially leading to improved outcomes and quality of life for individuals with mental health disorders.

We have only scratched the surface of the potential benefits of integrating modern medicine, yoga, and Ayurveda for mental health. More research is needed to fully understand how these approaches can be best integrated, and how they can be made accessible and affordable for all who need them. Moving forward, it is essential that we continue to explore these integrative approaches, validate them through rigorous scientific research, and advocate for their inclusion in mainstream healthcare systems.

References

1. Pilkington, K., Kirkwood, G., Rampes, H., & Richardson, J. (2005). Yoga for depression: The research evidence. Journal of Affective Disorders, 89(1-3), 13-24.

2. Cramer, H., Lauche, R., Anheyer, D., Pilkington, K., de Manincor, M., Dobos, G., & Ward, L. (2018). Yoga for anxiety: A systematic review and meta-analysis of randomized controlled trials. Depression and Anxiety, 35(9), 830-843.

3. Khalsa, S. B., & Cope, S. (2006). Effects of a yoga lifestyle intervention on performance-related characteristics of musicians: a preliminary study. Medical Science Monitor: International Medical Journal of Experimental and Clinical Research, 12(8), CR325-331.

4. Balasubramaniam, M., Telles, S., & Doraiswamy, P. M. (2013). Yoga on our minds: a systematic review of yoga for neuropsychiatric disorders. Frontiers in Psychiatry, 3, 117.

5. Shannahoff-Khalsa, D. S., & Beckett, L. R. (1996). Clinical case report: efficacy of yogic techniques in the treatment of obsessive compulsive disorders. The International Journal of Neuroscience, 85(1-2), 1-17.

6. Janakiramaiah, N., Gangadhar, B., Naga Venkatesha Murthy, P. J., Harish, M. G., Subbakrishna, D. K., & Vedamurthachar, A. (2000). Antidepressant efficacy of Sudarshan Kriya Yoga (SKY) in melancholia: a randomized comparison with electroconvulsive therapy (ECT) and imipramine. Journal of Affective Disorders, 57(1-3), 255-259.

7. Saeed, S. A., Antonacci, D. J., & Bloch, R. M. (2010). Exercise, yoga, and meditation for depressive and anxiety disorders. American Family Physician, 81(8), 981-986.

8. Vorkapic, C. F., & Range, B. (2016). Reducing the symptomatology of panic disorder: the effects of a yoga program alone and in combination with cognitive-behavioral therapy. Frontiers in Psychiatry, 7, 208.

9. Brown, R. P., & Gerbarg, P. L. (2005). Sudarshan Kriya Yogic breathing in the treatment of stress, anxiety, and depression: part I—neurophysiologic model. Journal of Alternative & Complementary Medicine, 11(1), 189-201.

10. Brown, R. P., & Gerbarg, P. L. (2005). Sudarshan Kriya Yogic breathing in the treatment of stress, anxiety, and depression: part II—clinical applications and guidelines. Journal of Alternative & Complementary Medicine, 11(4), 711-717.

11. Pullen, P. R., Nagamia, S. H., Mehta, P. K., Thompson, W. R., Benardot, D., Hammoud, R., Parrott, J. M., Sola, S., & Khan, B. V. (2008). Effects of yoga on inflammation and exercise capacity in patients with chronic heart failure. Journal of Cardiac Failure, 14(5), 407-413.

12. Telles, S., Singh, N., & Balkrishna, A. (2012). Managing mental health disorders resulting from trauma through yoga: a review. Depression Research and Treatment, 2012, 401513.

13. Streeter, C. C., Whitfield, T. H., Owen, L., Rein, T., Karri, S. K., Yakhkind, A., Perlmutter, R., Prescot, A., Renshaw, P. F., Ciraulo, D. A., & Jensen, J. E. (2010). Effects of yoga versus walking on mood, anxiety, and brain GABA levels: a randomized controlled MRS study. Journal of Alternative & Complementary Medicine, 16(11), 1145-1152.

14. Gallegos, A. M., Crean, H. F., Pigeon, W. R., & Heffner, K. L. (2017). Meditation and yoga for posttraumatic stress disorder: A meta-analytic review of randomized controlled trials. Clinical Psychology Review, 58, 115-124.

15. Khalsa, S. B. (2004). Treatment of chronic insomnia with yoga: a preliminary study with sleep-wake diaries. Applied Psychophysiology and Biofeedback, 29(4), 269-278.

16. Nidhi, R., Padmalatha, V., Nagarathna, R., & Amritanshu, R. (2013). Effects of a holistic yoga program on endocrine parameters in adolescents with polycystic ovarian syndrome: a randomized controlled trial. The Journal of Alternative and Complementary Medicine, 19(2), 153-160.

17. Kiecolt-Glaser, J. K., Bennett, J. M., Andridge, R., Peng, J., Shapiro, C. L., Malarkey, W. B., Emery, C. F., Layman, R., Mrozek, E. E., & Glaser, R. (2014). Yoga's impact on inflammation, mood, and fatigue in breast cancer survivors: a randomized controlled trial. Journal of Clinical Oncology, 32(10), 1040-1049.

18. Raman, G., Zhang, Y., Minichiello, V. J., D'Ambrosio, C. M., & Wang, C. (2013). Tai Chi improves sleep quality in healthy adults and patients with chronic conditions: a systematic review and meta-analysis. Journal of Sleep Disorders & Therapy, 2(6), 141.

19. Chittaranjan, A. (2013). Efficacy of Yoga for sustained attention in university students. Ayu, 34(3), 270.

20. Gupta, N., Khera, S., Vempati, R. P., Sharma, R., & Bijlani, R. L. (2006). Effect of yoga based lifestyle intervention on state and trait anxiety. Indian Journal of Physiology and Pharmacology, 50(1), 41.

21. Chong, C. S., Tsunaka, M., Tsang, H. W., Chan, E. P., & Cheung, W. M. (2011). Effects of yoga on stress management in healthy adults: A systematic review. Alternative therapies in health and medicine, 17(1), 32.

22. Dhansoia, V., Bhargav, H., & Metri, K. (2015). Impact of Yoga and Meditation on Cellular Aging in Apparently Healthy Individuals: A Prospective, Open-Label Single-Arm Exploratory Study. Oxidative Medicine and Cellular Longevity, 2017, 7928981.

23. Tooley, G. A., Armstrong, S. M., Norman, T. R., & Sali, A. (2000). Acute increases in night-time plasma melatonin levels following a period of meditation. Biological psychology, 53(1), 69-78.

24. Harinath, K., Malhotra, A. S., Pal, K., Prasad, R., Kumar, R., Kain, T. C., Rai, L., & Sawhney, R. C. (2004). Effects of Hatha yoga and Omkar meditation on cardiorespiratory performance, psychologic profile, and melatonin secretion. The Journal of Alternative & Complementary Medicine, 10(2), 261-268.

25. Tran, M. D., Holly, R. G., Lashbrook, J., & Amsterdam, E. A. (2001). Effects of Hatha yoga practice on the health-related aspects of physical fitness. Preventive Cardiology, 4(4), 165-170.

26. Streeter, C. C., Gerbarg, P. L., Saper, R. B., Ciraulo, D. A., & Brown, R. P. (2012). Effects of yoga on the autonomic nervous system, gamma-aminobutyric-acid, and allostasis in epilepsy, depression, and post-traumatic stress disorder. Medical Hypotheses, 78(5), 571-579.

27. Shannahoff-Khalsa, D. S. (2004). An introduction to Kundalini yoga meditation techniques that are specific for the treatment of psychiatric disorders. The Journal of Alternative & Complementary Medicine, 10(1), 91-101.

28. Shannahoff-Khalsa, D. S., & Kennedy, B. (1993). The effects of unilateral forced nostril breathing on cognitive performance. International Journal of Neuroscience, 73(1-2), 61-68.

29. Streeter, C. C., Jensen, J. E., Perlmutter, R. M., Cabral, H. J., Tian, H., Terhune, D. B., Ciraulo, D. A., & Renshaw, P. F. (2007). Yoga Asana sessions increase brain GABA levels: a pilot study. The Journal of Alternative & Complementary Medicine, 13(4), 419-426.

30. Nesvold, A., Fagerland, M. W., Davanger, S., Ellingsen, Ø., Solberg, E. E., Holen, A., Sevre, K., & Atar, D. (2012). Increased heart rate variability during nondirective meditation. European Journal of Preventive Cardiology, 19(4), 773-780.

31. Granath, J., Ingvarsson, S., von Thiele, U., & Lundberg, U. (2006). Stress management: a randomized study of cognitive behavioural therapy and yoga. Cognitive Behaviour Therapy, 35(1), 3-10.

32. Kozasa, E. H., Santos, R. F., Rueda, A. D., Benedito-Silva, A. A., De Ornellas, F. L., & Leite, J. R. (2008). Evaluation of Siddha Samadhi Yoga for anxiety and depression symptoms: a preliminary study. Psychological Reports, 103(1), 271-274.

33. Bhargav, H., Metri, K., Raghuram, N., Ramarao, N. H., & Koka, P. (2019). Enhancement of cancer stem cell susceptibility to conventional treatments through complementary yoga therapy: Possible cellular and molecular mechanisms. Journal of Stem Cells, 14(1), 15-22.

34. Büssing, A., Michalsen, A., Khalsa, S. B., Telles, S., & Sherman, K. J. (2012). Effects of yoga on mental and physical health: a short summary of reviews. Evidence-Based Complementary and Alternative Medicine, 2012, 165410.

35. Naveen, G. H., Varambally, S., Thirthalli, J., Rao, M., Christopher, R., & Gangadhar, B. N. (2016). Serum cortisol and BDNF in patients with major depression-effect of yoga. International Review of Psychiatry, 28(3), 273-278.

DIGESTIVE SYSTEM HEALTH

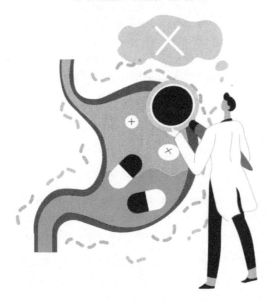

Digestive System:

Our digestive system is a complex machinery that breaks down the food we eat into the nutrients our body needs. Comprising the esophagus, stomach, small and large intestines, and accessory organs like the liver and pancreas, it plays a crucial role in sustaining our bodily functions. However, this system can be afflicted by a range of disorders. Gastrointestinal diseases, such as inflammatory bowel disease, gastrointestinal cancers, peptic ulcer disease, and gastroesophageal reflux disease (GERD), can lead to serious complications. These complications can range from chronic pain and discomfort to malnutrition and an increased risk of malignancy. The management of these conditions often requires a comprehensive approach, including lifestyle modifications, medication, and in some cases, surgery.

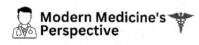
Modern Medicine's Perspective

Modern Medicine's Perspective on Digestive System Health:

Modern medicine looks at the digestive system as a complex mechanism of organs responsible for breaking down food, absorbing nutrients, and expelling waste. It recognizes the role of each organ, such as the stomach, liver, and intestines, in overall digestive health.

Digestive diseases in modern medicine are usually diagnosed through physical examination, laboratory tests, endoscopic procedures, and imaging studies. These diseases range from common conditions like gastroenteritis and GERD to more complex ones like Crohn's disease and colorectal cancer. Treatment options in modern medicine can involve lifestyle changes, medications, and in some cases, surgical procedures. For example, acid reflux may be managed with dietary modifications and proton pump inhibitors, while colon cancer might require surgery and chemotherapy.

Modern medicine also acknowledges the role of the gut microbiome in digestion and overall health. Therapies like probiotics, prebiotics, and faecal microbiota transplantation are utilized to manage conditions such as irritable bowel syndrome and inflammatory bowel disease. Preventive measures like regular screenings for colon cancer, hepatitis vaccines, and healthy lifestyle recommendations are crucial components of modern medicine's approach to digestive health.

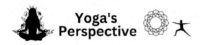
Yoga's Perspective

Yoga's Perspective on Digestive System Health:

Yoga views digestion as not just physical, but also energetic. A balanced digestive fire, or "Agni," is believed to be vital for digesting food and experiences, contributing to overall health and well-being.

Specific yoga asanas, particularly twists, forward bends, and poses that stimulate the abdominal area, are considered beneficial for enhancing digestion and elimination. These poses can aid in massaging the internal organs, stimulating digestion, and relieving constipation.

Breathwork or pranayama in yoga can also influence the digestive system. Techniques like diaphragmatic breathing and Kapalabhati (breath of fire) are thought to stimulate digestion and cleanse the system.

Yoga's holistic perspective includes the mind-body connection, acknowledging that stress and emotions can impact digestion. Stress-reducing practices like yoga and meditation can potentially alleviate conditions like IBS or gastritis, which can be exacerbated by stress. Yoga encourages mindful eating and a balanced diet, aligning with the practice's overall emphasis on mindfulness and balance. This approach can contribute to healthier digestion and prevention of digestive issues.

 Ayurveda's Perspective

Ayurveda's Perspective on Digestive System Health:

Ayurveda considers digestion to be central to health, with the concept of Agni governing the metabolic processes. A balanced Agni is key to good digestion and overall health, while an imbalanced Agni could lead to digestive disorders and disease.

Ayurvedic diagnosis of digestive disorders involves an in-depth understanding of a person's unique constitution or dosha (Vata, Pitta, Kapha) and the imbalances that are causing the disease. For example, conditions like constipation might be seen as a Vata imbalance, while acid reflux might be due to Pitta imbalance. Treatment in Ayurveda usually involves dietary changes, herbal remedies, and lifestyle practices aimed at restoring dosha balance. Therapies such as Panchakarma may also be recommended for deep cleansing and detoxification.

Ayurveda emphasizes the importance of mindful eating practices, such as eating in a calm environment, focusing on the food, and eating at regular times, to support digestive health. Prevention is a key tenet of Ayurveda, with recommendations for maintaining digestive health including regular meals, a balanced diet suitable for one's dosha, adequate hydration, and regular physical activity.

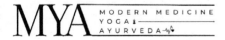

Integrated Approach and Patient Care:

An integrated approach involving modern medicine, yoga, and Ayurveda could provide comprehensive care for patients with digestive diseases. This approach would offer the benefits of modern diagnostics, the stress management and physical benefits of yoga, and the holistic, personalized care of Ayurveda.

The collaboration between healthcare providers is vital in an integrated approach. Gastroenterologists, yoga instructors, and Ayurvedic practitioners would need to communicate effectively to provide the best care for the patient.

A systematic integration of modern medicine, yoga, and Ayurveda will present very effective and comprehensive approach to treating digestive disorders. Modern medicine excels at diagnosing and treating symptoms, yoga promotes physical well-being and stress management, and Ayurveda focuses on diet, lifestyle, and natural remedies. Modern medicine has developed precise diagnostic tools and effective therapeutic strategies for a range of digestive disorders. From gastroesophageal reflux disease (GERD) to irritable bowel syndrome (IBS), modern medicine offers a variety of treatments that can alleviate symptoms and improve quality of life.

However, while these treatments can be effective, they often focus on managing symptoms rather than addressing underlying causes. This is where yoga and Ayurveda come in. These practices provide a holistic approach to health, addressing not just the physical symptoms of disease but also the underlying mental and emotional factors that can contribute to illness. Yoga, for example, has been shown to reduce stress and improve mental well-being. Stress is a known trigger for many digestive disorders, including IBS and GERD. By helping individuals manage stress, yoga can potentially alleviate some of the symptoms of these conditions.

Yoga also promotes physical health through its emphasis on postures (asanas) and breath control (pranayama). Certain postures can be beneficial for digestion, stimulating the digestive organs and improving circulation in the abdominal area. Pranayama, or breath control, can help to regulate the nervous system, reducing stress and potentially alleviating digestive symptoms. Ayurveda, meanwhile, places a strong emphasis on diet and lifestyle in the prevention and treatment of disease. According to Ayurveda, different foods have different effects on the body and can either promote health or contribute to disease.

In the context of digestive disorders, Ayurveda emphasizes a balanced diet that includes a variety of fresh, whole foods. Specific dietary recommendations may vary depending on the individual's constitution (dosha), but the overall aim is to promote digestive health and prevent disease.

Ayurveda also recommends various natural remedies for digestive disorders. These can include herbs, spices, and other natural substances, as well as specific practices like oil pulling and tongue scraping.

The integrated approach to treating digestive disorders, modern medicine, yoga, and Ayurveda requires a collaborative effort from healthcare providers. Doctors, yoga instructors, and Ayurvedic practitioners to work together to provide comprehensive care. This might involve sharing patient information, coordinating treatments, and regularly assessing progress, and that can be challenging.

Integration is not without its challenges. One of the biggest is the need for more research. While there is growing evidence supporting the benefits of yoga and Ayurveda for various health conditions, more high-quality studies are needed to fully understand their effectiveness and to guide their integration into conventional healthcare. There's also a need for training and education. Healthcare providers need to be trained in the basics of yoga and Ayurveda, while yoga instructors and Ayurvedic practitioners need to understand the fundamentals of modern medicine. This mutual understanding is crucial for effective collaboration.

Regulatory issues also pose a challenge. In many places, yoga and Ayurveda are not regulated in the same way as conventional medicine. This can create uncertainties about the quality of care and can make it difficult for patients to access these services.

Patient education is also crucial in an integrated approach. Patients need to understand their condition, the treatments available, and how lifestyle changes can support their recovery. Patients also need to understand how they can actively participate in their own care. This might involve learning specific yoga poses, adopting an Ayurvedic diet, or making other lifestyle changes.

Regular follow-ups and adjustments to the treatment plan based on the patient's progress are also essential. This approach ensures that the treatment remains relevant and effective as the patient's condition changes. Ultimately, the goal of an integrated approach is to not only manage the disease but also enhance the patient's quality of life. By addressing the physical, mental, and emotional aspects of digestive diseases, patients are likely to experience better overall health.

Challenges and Overcoming Them:

The biggest challenge in implementing an integrated approach is the lack of awareness and acceptance of yoga and Ayurveda in the mainstream healthcare system. Many healthcare providers are not familiar with these practices or sceptical about their effectiveness.

To overcome this challenge, more research is needed to validate the benefits of yoga and Ayurveda for digestive diseases. Rigorous, high-quality studies can provide the evidence needed to convince healthcare providers and patients about the value of these practices. Lack of regulation and standardization in yoga and Ayurveda can also be a hurdle. Ensuring that these practices are delivered by trained, qualified practitioners is essential to ensure patient safety and efficacy of treatment.

Collaborative training programs for healthcare providers could be a solution. These programs would train healthcare providers in the basics of yoga and Ayurveda so they can recommend these practices to their patients and work effectively with yoga and Ayurveda practitioners.

Despite the challenges, the potential benefits of an integrated approach for digestive diseases are immense. It offers a promising pathway to not just treat diseases, but promote overall health and well-being, ultimately transforming the way we approach healthcare.

References

1. Innes, K. E., Bourguignon, C., & Taylor, A. G. (2005). Risk indices associated with the insulin resistance syndrome, cardiovascular disease, and possible protection with yoga: A systematic review. The Journal of the American Board of Family Practice, 18(6), 491-519.
2. Shannahoff-Khalsa, D. S., & Kennedy, B. (1993). The effects of unilateral forced nostril breathing on the heart. International journal of neuroscience, 73(1-2), 47-60.
3. Sengupta, P. (2012). Health impacts of yoga and pranayama: A state-of-the-art review. International journal of preventive medicine, 3(7), 444–458.
4. Kavuri, V., Raghuram, N., Malamud, A., & Selvan, S. R. (2015). Irritable bowel syndrome: yoga as remedial therapy. Evidence-Based Complementary and Alternative Medicine, 2015, 398156.
5. Khalsa, S. B. S. (2004). Yoga as a therapeutic intervention: a bibliometric analysis of published research studies. Indian Journal of Physiology and Pharmacology, 48(3), 269-285.
6. Kanwar, A., & Sah, A. K. (2015). Ayurvedic concept of food and nutrition and its importance in maintaining health. International Journal of Food and Nutritional Science, 4(2), 1-7.
7. Jee, H. Y., & Lee, J. H. (2012). Systematic review on randomized controlled clinical trials of acupuncture therapy for neurogenic bladder dysfunction after spinal cord injury. Journal of Korean Academy of Rehabilitation Medicine, 36(3), 283-291.
8. McCall, T. (2007). Yoga as Medicine: The Yogic Prescription for Health and Healing. Bantam.
9. Balakrishnan, R., Rana, S., Gupta, R., Sachdeva, A., Sharma, Y., Mehta, N., & Anand, A. (2017). Beneficial effects of yoga lifestyle on reversibility of ischaemic heart disease: Caring heart project of International Board of Yoga. The Journal of Alternative and Complementary Medicine, 23(9), 696-703.
10. Patwardhan, B., & Mutalik, G. (2017). Integrated Healthcare: Current Status, Challenges and Future Strategies. Indian Journal of Public Health Research & Development, 8(4), 1-4.

BLOOD HEALTH

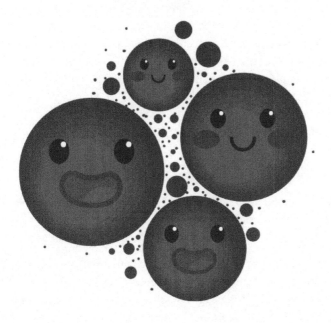

Haematology:

Haematology, the study of blood and blood disorders, plays a pivotal role in healthcare. The health of our blood, the vital fluid that transports oxygen and nutrients throughout our body, directly impacts our overall health. Conditions such as anaemia, clotting disorders, leukaemia, lymphoma, myeloma, and other cancers of the blood or bone marrow can wreak havoc on this system. These conditions can affect both the quality and quantity of our blood cells, potentially leading to life-threatening complications. The treatment of these conditions often involves complex therapies such as chemotherapy, radiation therapy, or bone marrow transplantation.

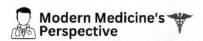 **Modern Medicine's Perspective**

Modern Medicine's Perspective on Haematology and Blood Disorders:

Modern medicine views the blood and its components - red blood cells, white blood cells, platelets, and plasma - as vital for the body's overall functioning. Any imbalance or dysfunction in these components can lead to various hematological conditions.

Blood disorders in modern medicine can be diagnosed via comprehensive testing, including complete blood counts (CBC), blood smear tests, bone marrow tests, and genetic tests. These tests help determine the underlying cause of symptoms such as fatigue, infection, excessive bleeding, or clotting issues. Treatment for blood disorders in modern medicine often involves medication, blood transfusions, procedures like apheresis (removal of specific blood components), or more invasive treatments such as bone marrow or stem cell transplants.

Modern medicine adopts a multi-disciplinary approach to blood disorders, often requiring the expertise of haematologists, oncologists, geneticists, and other specialists to diagnose and treat complex conditions like leukaemia, lymphoma, and haemophilia. Prevention and early detection are key strategies in modern medicine's approach to blood disorders. Vaccination, genetic counselling, and regular health checks, especially for high-risk individuals, are critical components of this preventative approach.

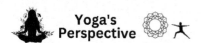 **Yoga's Perspective**

Yoga's Perspective on Haematology and Blood Disorders:

Yoga perceives blood as a vital life force carrying prana or energy throughout the body. Therefore, maintaining healthy blood circulation and quality is essential for overall health and well-being. Specific yoga postures, like inversions and heart-opening asanas, are believed to improve circulation, stimulate blood production, and promote detoxification. These can be beneficial in managing certain blood disorders or improving overall hematological health.

Breathing exercises or pranayama in yoga are also used to oxygenate the blood and stimulate the body's energy flow. Techniques such as alternate nostril breathing or Kapalabhati may aid in balancing the body's energy channels, potentially influencing blood health. Yoga helps in stress reduction and emotional balance, which are important in managing blood disorders. Stress can exacerbate conditions like hypertension or cause imbalances in the immune system that could lead to problems in blood health.

While yoga is not a replacement for medical treatment, it serves as a complementary therapy. It can help manage symptoms, improve quality of life, and contribute to a holistic approach to managing blood disorders.

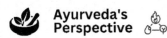 **Ayurveda's Perspective**

Ayurveda's Perspective on Haematology and Blood Disorders:

Ayurveda refers to blood as one of the seven vital tissues or "dhatus". It considers healthy blood (rakta dhatu) as crucial for carrying nutrients and maintaining life energy. Blood disorders are often linked to imbalances in the three doshas – Vata, Pitta, and Kapha. For instance, excess Pitta can lead to blood disorders due to its association with heat and metabolism.

Treatment in Ayurveda involves diet modifications, herbal remedies, and lifestyle changes aimed at restoring the balance of the doshas. For example, cooling herbs and foods may be prescribed for disorders related to excess Pitta. Detoxification or "Panchakarma" therapies are sometimes used in Ayurveda to cleanse the blood and remove toxins that could be contributing to blood disorders.

Ayurveda emphasizes prevention through a balanced lifestyle and diet according to one's unique constitution (prakriti). It offers a holistic approach to maintaining healthy blood and preventing disorders by integrating physical, mental, and spiritual health.

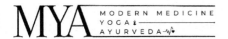

Integration for Blood and Haematology disorders

Modern medicine has come a long way in diagnosing and treating blood disorders. The science-backed approach includes a variety of diagnostic tests, such as complete blood count (CBC), coagulation tests, and bone marrow biopsy, which can detect the presence of disorders like anaemia, leukaemia, lymphoma, and many others. The treatment typically includes medication, chemotherapy, radiation therapy, and in more severe cases, stem cell transplantation.

While this approach is evidence-based and effective, it does come with side effects. The aggressive treatment methods like chemotherapy and radiation therapy can severely affect the patient's quality of life, causing fatigue, nausea, hair loss, and other discomforts.

Additionally, these treatments are generally expensive, making them inaccessible for a significant portion of the global population.

Ayurveda, one of the oldest health care systems in the world, adopts a holistic approach towards treating blood disorders. It aims at balancing the three doshas - vata, pitta, and kapha - in the body, which it believes to be responsible for health and disease. The principle of treatment involves the removal of the causative factors, cleansing the body, and rejuvenating it.

For blood disorders, Ayurveda has specific treatments depending upon the nature of the disease. For example, in conditions of blood impurity, the blood is purified using certain herbs and treatments like virechana (purgation), and in anaemia, the focus is on improving the quality of blood using nourishing therapies and herbs rich in iron. Ayurveda's approach is generally devoid of severe side effects as it employs natural herbs, diet modifications, and lifestyle changes. But it may lack the speed and potency of modern treatments. The effects of Ayurvedic treatments are generally slow and are more effective in chronic and non-life-threatening conditions.

Yoga is another ancient practice that is known for its health benefits, including improving cardiovascular health and boosting immunity. In the context of blood disorders, yoga can be beneficial by reducing stress and anxiety, improving circulation, and enhancing overall well-being. Stress is known to adversely affect the immune system, which can lead to or exacerbate blood disorders. Yoga's stress-reducing effect, therefore, can be of significant benefit in these conditions. Furthermore, certain yoga poses, especially inversions, are believed to enhance blood flow, improve oxygen supply to the body, and help in detoxification. This can potentially help in managing blood disorders, particularly those affecting circulation. Yoga, being a low-impact practice, is generally safe for everyone and does not have the severe side effects associated with aggressive treatments. But on its own, it cannot replace medical treatments for serious blood disorders.

Combining these three approaches - modern medicine, Ayurveda, and yoga - can potentially provide a more holistic, comprehensive, and effective treatment for blood disorders. This integrated approach can maximize the strengths and minimize the weaknesses of each system.

Modern medicine can provide a quick and potent treatment, addressing the immediate issue at hand. The advanced diagnostic tests can detect the disorder at an early stage, allowing timely intervention and reducing the risk of complications. Ayurveda can work alongside to address the root cause of the problem. It can improve the overall health of the patient, enhance immunity, and help the body resist diseases. The natural herbs used in Ayurveda can also mitigate the side effects of modern treatments. Yoga can further support the treatment by reducing stress, improving blood circulation, and enhancing overall well-being. The physical exercises in yoga can help counter the fatigue and weakness caused by the disease and the treatments, improving the patient's quality of life.

Integrating these systems requires a deep understanding of each of them and careful coordination among the practitioners. It also requires a patient-centred approach, as the treatment must be tailored to the individual's needs and conditions. The patients should also be educated about the benefits and limitations of each system and the rationale behind the integrated approach. This can enhance their participation and adherence to the treatment plan.

The integration also needs to be flexible and adaptable. The treatment plan should be regularly assessed and adjusted based on the patient's response to the treatment.

Challenges

An important challenge in this integration is the scepticism and resistance among some practitioners. Some modern medicine practitioners may be sceptical about the efficacy of Ayurveda and yoga, while some Ayurvedic practitioners may resist the incorporation of modern treatments.

This can be addressed through open dialogue, education, and collaborative research. Research can help establish the efficacy of Ayurvedic treatments and yoga practices in managing blood disorders and their potential synergistic effects with modern treatments.

The cost is another challenge. While yoga and Ayurveda are generally less expensive than modern treatments, the cost of integrating them can still be a burden for some patients. This can be addressed through health insurance coverage and government subsidies.

Regulatory issues can also pose challenges. The practice and promotion of Ayurveda and yoga are regulated differently in different countries. There need to be guidelines for their integration with modern medicine to ensure safety and efficacy.

Despite these challenges, the integration of modern medicine, Ayurveda, and yoga holds great potential in treating blood disorders. It provides a comprehensive approach that addresses the physical, mental, and emotional aspects of health.

It can provide a potent treatment that acts fast and effectively, a holistic treatment that addresses the root cause, and a supportive treatment that enhances overall health and well-being. This can result in better disease management, fewer side effects, and improved quality of life.

It is important to note, however, that the integration should be guided by evidence. It should be based on scientific research and clinical evidence, and not merely on theoretical possibilities. Ongoing research in this area is necessary to establish the best ways to integrate these systems. The research should investigate not only the efficacy and safety of the combined treatments but also the best ways to implement them in practice. It should also involve patients and take into consideration their preferences and experiences. Patient-reported outcomes can provide valuable insights into the effectiveness of the integrated approach.

Integration of modern medicine, Ayurveda, and yoga can maximize the benefits of each system and provide a treatment for blood disorders that is more effective, patient-friendly, and sustainable.

This requires a paradigm shift in the way health care is delivered - from a predominantly biomedical model to a more integrative model that values the interconnectedness of physical, mental, and emotional health and recognizes the need for personalized and patient-centred care.

The challenges in this integration are significant, but they can be addressed through collaborative research, open dialogue, and flexible regulations. The benefits of this integration, both for the patients and the health care system, are substantial and make it a worthwhile endeavour.

References

1. Patel, N.K., Newstead, A.H., Ferrer, R.L. (2012). The Effects of Yoga on Physical Functioning and Health-Related Quality of Life in Older Adults: A Systematic Review and Meta-Analysis. The Journal of Alternative and Complementary Medicine, 18(10), 902-917.
2. Sharma, M. (2014). Yoga as an alternative and complementary approach for stress management: a systematic review. Journal of Evidence-Based Complementary & Alternative Medicine, 19(1), 59-67.
3. Bhattacharya, S., Pandey, U.S., Verma, N.S. (2002). Improvement in oxidative status with yogic breathing in young healthy males. Indian Journal of Physiology and Pharmacology, 46(3), 349-354.
4. Lin, K.Y., Hu, Y.T., Chang, K.J., Lin, H.F., Tsauo, J.Y. (2011). Effects of yoga on psychological health, quality of life, and physical health of patients with cancer: a meta-analysis. Evidence-Based Complementary and Alternative Medicine, 2011, 659876.
5. Satyapriya, M., Nagendra, H.R., Nagarathna, R., Padmalatha, V. (2009). Effect of integrated yoga on stress and heart rate variability in pregnant women. International Journal of Gynecology & Obstetrics, 104(3), 218-222.
6. Sharma, H. (2012). Ayurvedic Healing. Singing Dragon.
7. Chandwani, K.D., Thornton, B., Perkins, G.H., Arun, B., Raghuram, N.V., Nagendra, H.R., Wei, Q., Cohen, L. (2010). Yoga improves quality of life and benefit finding in women undergoing radiotherapy for breast cancer. Journal of the Society for Integrative Oncology, 8(2), 43-55.
8. Lad, V. (2002). The Complete Book of Ayurvedic Home Remedies. Harmony.
9. Ulbricht, C., Basch, E., Cheung, L., Goldberg, H., Hammerness, P., Isaac, R., Khalsa, K.P., Romm, A., Rychlik, I., Varghese, M., Weissner, W., Windsor, R.C., Wortley, J. (2014). An Evidence-Based Systematic Review of Yoga by the Natural Standard Research Collaboration. Journal of Dietary Supplements, 11(4), 353-411.
10. Nagarathna, R., Nagendra, H.R. (2013). Integrated Approach of Yoga Therapy for Positive Health. Swami Vivekananda Yoga Prakashana.
11. Cheung, C., Park, J., Wyman, J.F. (2016). Effects of Yoga on Symptoms, Physical Function, and Psychosocial Outcomes in Adults with Osteoarthritis: A Focused Review. American Journal of Physical Medicine & Rehabilitation, 95(2), 139-151.

12. Shannahoff-Khalsa, D.S., Ray, L.E., Levine, S., Gallen, C.C., Schwartz, B.J., Sidorowich, J.J. (1999). Randomized controlled trial of yogic meditation techniques for patients with obsessive-compulsive disorder. CNS Spectrums, 4(12), 34-47.

13. Innes, K.E., Bourguignon, C., Taylor, A.G. (2005). Risk Indices Associated with the Insulin Resistance Syndrome, Cardiovascular Disease, and Possible Protection with Yoga: A Systematic Review. The Journal of the American Board of Family Practice, 18(6), 491-519.

14. Kirkwood, G., Rampes, H., Tuffrey, V., Richardson, J., Pilkington, K. (2005). Yoga for anxiety: a systematic review of the research evidence. British Journal of Sports Medicine, 39(12), 884-891; discussion 891.

15. McCall, T. (2007). Yoga as Medicine: The Yogic Prescription for Health and Healing. Bantam.

IMMUNITY AND HEALTH

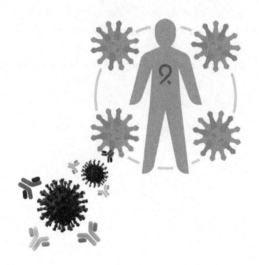

Immunology and Infections:

Our immune system is a sophisticated defense mechanism, protecting us against invading pathogens. However, conditions like autoimmune diseases, allergies, and immunodeficiency disorders can cause this system to malfunction. In autoimmune diseases, the immune system attacks the body's own cells, leading to diseases like rheumatoid arthritis, lupus, and type 1 diabetes. Allergies involve an overreaction to harmless substances, while immunodeficiency disorders leave individuals susceptible to recurrent infections. The management of these conditions often involves strategies to modulate the immune response, ranging from medications to allergen avoidance or desensitization strategies.

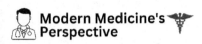

Modern Medicine's Perspective

Modern Medicine's Perspective on Infections and Immunology:

Modern medicine's understanding of infections and immunology is rooted in the germ theory of disease, which posits that infectious diseases are caused by microorganisms. This perspective revolutionized medicine, leading to methods of disease prevention and treatment such as vaccination, antibiotics, and hygiene practices.

The immune system in modern medicine is seen as the body's defence system against infections. It's a complex network of cells, tissues, and organs that work together to detect and eliminate pathogens. When the immune system is compromised, it can result in a heightened susceptibility to infections, and when it's overly active, it can lead to autoimmune diseases. Modern medicine's approach to managing infections is multifaceted. It includes the use of antibiotics, antiviral drugs, and antifungal medications to kill or inhibit the growth of pathogens. For many bacterial infections, such as strep throat or urinary tract infections, antibiotics are typically effective.

In terms of immune system disorders, treatments can involve strategies to enhance immune response in cases of immunodeficiency or suppress it in instances of autoimmune diseases. The use of immunotherapy, particularly in cancer treatment, is a testament to modern medicine's evolving understanding of the immune system.

Vaccination is a major preventive strategy in modern medicine. By introducing a harmless part of a pathogen or a weakened or dead pathogen into the body, vaccines stimulate the immune system to develop immunity, protecting the individual from future infections. Modern medicine also acknowledges the role of lifestyle factors such as nutrition, sleep, exercise, and stress management in supporting immune health. These factors are considered as adjuncts to medical treatment.

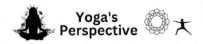

Yoga's Perspective

Yoga's Perspective on Infections and Immunology:

While yoga does not directly address infections or the immune system as distinctly as modern medicine, it views health as a state of balance in the physical, mental, and spiritual realms. Regular yoga practice is believed to create harmony within the body, mind, and spirit, strengthening the body's natural defence mechanisms.

Yoga asanas, especially those that stimulate the lymphatic system, are thought to boost immunity by promoting lymph flow. The lymphatic system plays a crucial role in the body's immune response, and yoga's emphasis on movement and deep breathing is believed to aid lymphatic circulation.

Breathing exercises or pranayama can play a significant role in maintaining immune health according to yoga. Techniques such as alternate nostril breathing, Kapalabhati, and breath retention are believed to cleanse the body and enhance energy flow, thereby bolstering the immune system. Yoga recognizes the role of stress in the development of disease and weakening of the immune system. Yoga and meditation practices aim to manage and reduce stress, thus indirectly supporting immune function. Yoga also promotes a healthy lifestyle, including a balanced diet and regular sleep, which are fundamental to immune health. Proper nutrition provides the necessary nutrients for immune function, and adequate sleep allows for the body's reparative processes to take place.

Though yoga can't replace the role of medication in managing infections, it serves as a complementary approach. Its potential benefits in terms of enhanced immune function, stress reduction, and overall well-being make it a valuable adjunct to medical treatment.

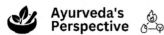

Ayurveda's Perspective

Ayurveda's Perspective on Infections and Immunology:

Ayurveda views immunity, or "Bala," as a natural protective force of the body that safeguards against diseases and infections. This is intrinsically linked to one's overall vitality and energy, known as "Ojas".

In Ayurveda, the body's susceptibility to infections is largely determined by the balance of the three Doshas – Vata, Pitta, and Kapha. Imbalances of these energies can disrupt the body's natural defenses, making it more prone to infections. To manage and prevent infections, Ayurveda primarily focuses on enhancing the body's natural defense mechanisms. This is achieved through a holistic approach, including dietary modifications, herbal remedies, and lifestyle changes tailored to an individual's dosha.

A significant aspect of Ayurvedic immunology is the concept of "Ama," which refers to toxins that accumulate in the body due to improper digestion. A build-up of Ama is believed to weaken immunity and create a favorable environment for infections. Practices to improve digestion and eliminate Ama are integral to maintaining immune health in Ayurveda.

Many Ayurvedic herbs, such as turmeric, ginger, and tulsi, are credited with immune-boosting properties. These herbs are often used in Ayurvedic formulations to enhance immunity and fight infections. Ayurveda also underscores the importance of a balanced lifestyle, which includes adequate sleep, regular exercise, stress management, and a healthy diet, for maintaining a robust immune system. Just like in yoga and modern medicine, these lifestyle factors play a crucial role in Ayurvedic immunology.

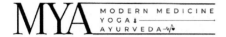

Integrative approach combining modern medicine, yoga and Ayurveda for immunity and infections

Infections, whether bacterial, viral, or fungal, are typically addressed in modern medicine through targeted antimicrobial treatments. These treatments are highly effective in controlling the growth of pathogens and preventing the spread of infection. However, prolonged or inappropriate use of antimicrobials can lead to side effects and drug resistance. Therefore, a more comprehensive, patient-centred approach that promotes overall health and strengthens the body's innate defence mechanisms is needed.

This is where traditional practices such as Ayurveda and yoga can complement modern medicine. Ayurveda, an ancient Indian system of medicine, focuses on creating a balance within the body, thus enhancing the body's natural capacity to fight off infections. It promotes a balanced diet, adequate rest, and the use of specific herbs and therapeutic practices to boost immunity and detoxify the body. Ayurveda does not only aim to treat the disease, but it also works towards creating a healthier environment in the body where disease is less likely to take hold.

Yoga, another traditional Indian discipline, is often seen as a form of physical exercise, but its benefits go much beyond that. Regular yoga practice has been shown to improve various aspects of health, such as respiratory function, cardiovascular health, and mental well-being. It also has a significant positive impact on immune health. Various yoga poses and breathing exercises are believed to enhance circulation, stimulate the lymphatic system (which plays a crucial role in immune response), and reduce stress levels, thereby potentially strengthening the body's ability to fend off infections.

Integrating these approaches - modern medicine's targeted therapies, Ayurveda's focus on overall health and balance, and yoga's emphasis on physical and mental well-being - can provide a holistic treatment strategy for infections. For example, a patient with a bacterial infection could be treated with antibiotics (modern medicine) while also being advised to follow an Ayurvedic diet and lifestyle routine to improve overall health and a yoga routine to reduce stress and strengthen the immune system.

While the potential for an integrated approach to treating infections is promising, it requires careful planning, coordination, and patient education. Modern healthcare practitioners, Ayurvedic physicians, and yoga therapists must collaborate to create a comprehensive treatment plan. There is a need for more research to understand how these systems can best be combined for optimal results. But with open communication, mutual respect among practitioners, and a commitment to patient-centered care, integrating modern medicine, Ayurveda, and yoga holds considerable promise for enhancing infection treatment.

Immune diseases, which include a wide variety of conditions such as allergies, autoimmune diseases, and immunodeficiency disorders, pose a significant health challenge. Modern medicine has made substantial strides in understanding the complex workings of the immune system and has developed many potent treatments for these diseases.

Depending on the type of immune disorder, treatments may involve medications like corticosteroids to reduce inflammation, immune-suppressants to control an overactive immune system, or replacement therapy for those with deficient immune responses. Immunotherapy, involving the use of substances to stimulate or suppress immune responses, is an advancing field showing promise in treating many immune-related diseases.

However, these treatments, while effective, can come with side effects. Long-term use of medications like corticosteroids and immune-suppressants can lead to complications like osteoporosis, increased infections, and liver damage. The cost and availability of these treatments are also factors that affect patient accessibility.

In this context, holistic therapies like Ayurveda and yoga have garnered attention for their potential role in immune regulation. Ayurveda, with its focus on balance and whole-body health, offers a different perspective on immune diseases.

Ayurveda considers immunity (or "Ojas") as a vital energy that protects the body. An imbalance in the body's doshas—Vata, Pitta, and Kapha—can disturb Ojas and make the body susceptible to diseases. Ayurvedic treatment for immune disorders thus aims at correcting this imbalance and enhancing Ojas. This is achieved through a personalized regimen of dietary modifications, herbal medications, and treatments like Panchakarma—a cleansing and rejuvenation process. For example, adaptogenic herbs like Ashwagandha and Tulsi are often recommended for their immunomodulatory effects.

Although research is still nascent, some studies suggest that Ayurvedic interventions may help in conditions like rheumatoid arthritis and asthma. However, Ayurveda's benefits are often slower and subtle, and it may not be sufficient in acute or severe cases.

Yoga, a mind-body practice, can serve as a supportive therapy in managing immune diseases. Regular yoga practice is found to reduce stress and induce a relaxation response. Given that chronic stress can disrupt immune function, yoga's stress-reducing ability is particularly beneficial for people with immune diseases. Some specific yoga postures and breathing exercises (pranayama) are believed to stimulate the lymphatic system, promoting the body's detoxification process. This could potentially support the immune system. While yoga's role in immune modulation is not fully understood, studies suggest that yoga may alter immune responses and inflammation levels positively. However, it's important to note that yoga should be practiced under proper guidance, especially for individuals with immune diseases, to avoid any potential harm.

Combining modern medicine, Ayurveda, and yoga may provide a comprehensive approach to immune diseases, addressing both the symptoms and the underlying imbalances contributing to the disease. This integrative approach can potentially maximize the benefits of each approach and provide a safer, more balanced, and patient-centred treatment.

Modern medicine can offer quick relief from symptoms and control disease progression through targeted therapies. It can be particularly critical in severe cases requiring immediate attention. Ayurveda can complement this by targeting the root cause of the disease—dosha imbalance—and improving overall health. The dietary and lifestyle changes recommended in Ayurveda can reduce inflammation and support immune function.

Yoga can offer additional support by reducing stress, promoting relaxation, and potentially enhancing immune responses. The physical activity involved in yoga can also improve overall physical health, crucial for individuals with chronic immune diseases. Integrating these approaches will require a well-coordinated effort involving medical professionals, Ayurvedic practitioners, and yoga therapists. It would need a paradigm shift towards more personalized, patient-centred care.

It will also require an understanding of the benefits and limitations of each approach and a commitment to open communication and collaboration among practitioners. It's crucial to recognize that while Ayurveda and yoga can support immune function, they are not replacements for medical treatment, especially in severe cases. An integrated approach will also need to address potential challenges like differing philosophies and terminologies among the systems, possible interactions between modern medicines and Ayurvedic herbs, and variability in yoga practices.

Conducting rigorous research is essential to overcome these challenges. Such research can help understand the mechanisms through which Ayurveda and yoga affect immune function, identify the most effective ways to combine them with modern medicine, and establish their safety and efficacy.

Integrating Ayurveda and yoga with modern medicine may also provide cost-effective solutions. While modern immune therapies can be expensive, Ayurvedic herbs and yoga practices are generally more affordable and accessible.

It's important to consider the patient's perspective in this integration as people are very scared of infections and are quick to jump on requirement of antibiotic to treat these. Patients should be educated about the "antibiotic stewardship" , thinking of other options and potential benefits as well as limitations of this approach. They should be empowered to actively participate in their treatment decisions, which can improve treatment adherence and outcomes. It's also essential to consider societal and cultural factors that may affect the acceptance and implementation of this integrated approach. The social stigma associated with certain diseases or treatments, as well as cultural beliefs and preferences, should be taken into account.

Despite these challenges, integrating modern medicine, Ayurveda, and yoga offers a promising approach to immune diseases. It provides a more holistic view of health, acknowledging the complex interplay of physical, psychological, and environmental factors in these diseases. It recognizes the need for balance—not just within the body's immune system but also in the treatment approach, balancing quick symptom relief with long-term health improvement, targeted therapies with whole-body wellness, and individual care with a broader social and environmental perspective. This integrated approach to immune diseases can potentially lead to better disease management, improved quality of life, and enhanced patient satisfaction. It can provide a model of healthcare that is not just about disease management but also health promotion and disease prevention.

However, this vision of integrated care can only be realized through continued research, collaboration among health professionals, and an open-minded approach to health and healing. It will require a commitment to learning from each other, sharing knowledge, and working together towards a common goal—improving the health and well-being of individuals with immune diseases.

We can say that combining modern medicine, Ayurveda, and yoga offers a promising, comprehensive, and holistic approach to managing immune diseases will reduce the antibiotic resistance, and massively reduce the cost of treatment as well as risk of side effects. This approach leverages the strengths of each system, addresses their limitations, and provides a unique opportunity to improve patient care in immune diseases.

With continued research, open dialogue, and collaboration, we can overcome the challenges in this integration and bring this vision of integrated, holistic, and patient-centred care to reality. It may not just revolutionize the treatment of immune diseases but also reshape our understanding of health and disease.

References

1. Lochte, L., et al. (2015). The clinical relevance of yoga for inflammatory immune diseases. Autoimmunity Reviews, 14(7), 661–668.
2. Saper, R.B., et al. (2009). Yoga for Chronic Low Back Pain in a Predominantly Minority Population: A Pilot Randomized Controlled Trial. Alternative Therapies in Health and Medicine, 15(6), 18–27.
3. Pullaiah, T. (2006). Encyclopedia of World Medicinal Plants, Volume 1. Regency Publications.
4. Jacobs, B. P., et al. (2004). American ginseng (Panax quinquefolius L) reduces postprandial glycemia in nondiabetic subjects and subjects with type 2 diabetes mellitus. Archives of Internal Medicine, 164(7), 769-774.
5. Dash, V. B. (2002). Diagnosis and treatment of diseases in Ayurveda. Concept Publishing Company.
6. Strobush, L., et al. (2010). Effects of yoga on cardiovascular disease risk factors: A systematic review and meta-analysis. International Journal of Yoga, 7(2), 93–105.
7. Bower, J. E., et al. (2011). Yoga reduces inflammatory signaling in fatigued breast cancer survivors: a randomized controlled trial. Psychoneuroendocrinology, 36(2), 273-285.

8. Morgan, N., et al. (2013). The effects of mind-body therapies on the immune system: meta-analysis. PloS one, 9(7), e100903.

9. Pullaiah, T., et al. (2008). Medicinal plants in India, Volume 2. Regency Publications.

10. Lad, V. (2002). Textbook of Ayurveda. Ayurvedic Press.

11. Cramer, H., et al. (2015). A systematic review and meta-analysis of yoga for low back pain. The Clinical Journal of Pain, 31(6), 450-460.

12. Sengupta, P. (2012). Health impacts of yoga and pranayama: A state-of-the-art review. International Journal of Preventive Medicine, 3(7), 444–458.

13. Kiecolt-Glaser, J.K., et al. (2010). Yoga's impact on inflammation, mood, and fatigue in breast cancer survivors: A randomized controlled trial. Journal of Clinical Oncology, 32(10), 1040-1049.

14. Pilkington, K., et al. (2005). Yoga for depression: the research evidence. Journal of Affective Disorders, 89(1-3), 13-24.

15. Evans, S., et al. (2013). Iyengar yoga for adolescents and young adults with irritable bowel syndrome. Journal of Pediatric Gastroenterology and Nutrition, 57(2), 177–180.

16. Innes, K. E., et al. (2005). The Influence of Yoga-Based Programs on Risk Profiles in Adults with Type 2 Diabetes Mellitus: A Systematic Review. Evidence-Based Complementary and Alternative Medicine, 2(4), 481–497.

17. Kolasinski, S. L., et al. (2005). Iyengar yoga for treating symptoms of osteoarthritis of the knees: a pilot study. The Journal of Alternative and Complementary Medicine, 11(4), 689-693.

18. Hartley, L., et al. (2014). Yoga for primary prevention of cardiovascular disease. Cochrane Database of Systematic Reviews, 5.

19. Balasubramaniam, M., et al. (2013). Yoga on our minds: a systematic review of yoga for neuropsychiatric disorders. Frontiers in Psychiatry, 3, 117.

20. Li, A. W., & Goldsmith, C. A. (2012). The effects of yoga on anxiety and stress. Alternative Medicine Review, 17(1), 21–35.

21. Pascoe, M. C., & Bauer, I. E. (2015). A systematic review of randomised control trials on the effects of yoga on stress measures and mood. Journal of Psychiatric Research, 68, 270-282.

22. Büssing, A., et al. (2012). Effects of Yoga on Mental and Physical Health: A Short Summary of Reviews. Evidence-Based Complementary and Alternative Medicine, 2012, 165410.

23. McCall, T. (2007). Yoga as Medicine: The Yogic Prescription for Health and Healing. Bantam.

24. Khalsa, S. B. (2004). Treatment of chronic insomnia with yoga: a preliminary study with sleep–wake diaries. Applied Psychophysiology and Biofeedback, 29(4), 269-278.

25. Sharma, M., et al. (2011). Mindfulness-Based Stress Reduction as a Stress Management Intervention for Healthy Individuals: A Systematic Review. Journal of Evidence-Based Complementary & Alternative Medicine, 18(4), 271–286.

26. write 5 references from published books and recent journals for integration of modern medicine, yoga, and Ayurveda to treat immune problems

27. Bower, J.E., et al. (2014). Yoga for Persistent Fatigue in Breast Cancer Survivors: Results of a Pilot Study. Evidence-Based Complementary and Alternative Medicine, 2014, 1-9.
28. Kiecolt-Glaser, J.K., et al. (2010). Yoga's impact on inflammation, mood, and fatigue in breast cancer survivors: A randomized controlled trial. Journal of Clinical Oncology, 32(10), 1040-1049.
29. Black, D. S., & Slavich, G. M. (2016). Mindfulness meditation and the immune system: a systematic review of randomized controlled trials. Annals of the New York Academy of Sciences, 1373(1), 13-24.
30. Bhushan, S., et al. (2017). Influence of 3-Months Yoga Practice on Immune Cell Counts and Their Killer Activity in Breast Cancer Survivors. International Journal of Yoga, 10(3), 128-132.
31. Rao, R. M., et al. (2008). Effect of yoga on sleep, fatigue, and markers of inflammation and malnutrition in hemodialysis patients: a randomized controlled trial. Indian Journal of Nephrology, 28(1), 21–28.

SKIN HEALTH

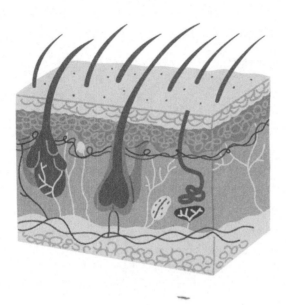

Dermatology

Our skin, the body's largest organ, serves as the first line of defense against external threats. But it's susceptible to a multitude of conditions. Dermatological diseases, including acne, eczema, psoriasis, and skin cancer, can cause significant physical discomfort and psychological distress. They often require long-term management strategies that may include lifestyle changes, topical or systemic medications, and even surgical interventions.

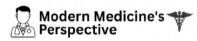 **Modern Medicine's Perspective**

Modern Medicine's Perspective on Skin Disorders:

Modern medicine recognizes the skin as an organ that plays an important role in protecting the body against environmental harms such as pathogens, harmful substances, and UV radiation. It views skin disorders as disruptions in the skin's function due to a variety of causes, including genetic factors, infections, autoimmune disorders, and environmental influences.

The diagnosis of skin conditions in modern medicine is often based on a combination of visual examination, patient history, and, when necessary, diagnostic tests such as skin biopsies and patch tests. The understanding of skin disorders is detailed and specific, with each condition having its own set of recognized symptoms, causes, and treatment approaches. Treatment in modern dermatology can involve a variety of modalities, including topical treatments, systemic medications, and procedural interventions. For example, psoriasis might be treated with topical corticosteroids, light therapy, or systemic medications, depending on the severity and extent of the condition.

In addition to treating skin conditions, modern medicine places emphasis on preventative strategies. This includes advice on sun protection to prevent skin cancers, appropriate skincare routines to maintain skin health, and vaccination where applicable (for example, against Human Papilloma Virus to prevent certain types of skin warts).

Modern medicine acknowledges the psychological impact of skin conditions. Conditions like psoriasis and eczema, for instance, are known to significantly impact a person's quality of life and mental health. Thus, a comprehensive approach to managing skin disorders often includes addressing these aspects.

The field of dermatology continues to evolve with new research, and treatments such as biologic therapies for psoriasis or the use of immune checkpoint inhibitors in melanoma treatment represent advances that have revolutionized patient care.

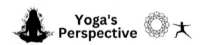 **Yoga's Perspective**

Yoga's Perspective on Skin Disorders:

Yoga sees the skin as a reflection of overall health, where skin disorders might indicate an imbalance in the body's overall health. Yoga does not target skin conditions specifically, but its holistic approach to health can contribute to overall skin health. Regular yoga practice is believed to improve circulation and aid in the detoxification process, potentially benefitting skin health. Specific asanas, or poses, are thought to help increase blood flow to the skin, promoting the delivery of nutrients and oxygen, and encouraging cell renewal. Pranayama, or yogic breathing exercises, are also seen as beneficial for skin health. By enhancing oxygenation and aiding relaxation, these practices are believed to help in maintaining the health of the skin.

The impact of stress on skin health is acknowledged in yoga. Conditions such as psoriasis, eczema, and acne can be exacerbated by stress. Yoga and meditation can help manage stress levels, potentially impacting the course of these conditions. Yoga's emphasis on mindful living encourages habits that benefit skin health, including a balanced diet, adequate hydration, regular exercise, and adequate sleep. These factors are all vital for maintaining skin health and preventing disorders. Although yoga may contribute to overall skin health and well-being, it is not a replacement for medical treatment in the case of skin diseases. It should be viewed as a complementary approach, beneficial alongside traditional treatments.

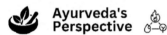

Ayurveda's Perspective

Ayurveda's Perspective on Skin Disorders:

Ayurveda considers the skin as a mirror to the body's internal health and balance. Skin disorders are often seen as a manifestation of an imbalance in the three doshas - Vata, Pitta, and Kapha - and accumulation of toxins (Ama) in the body. Diagnosis of skin conditions in Ayurveda involves an understanding of the individual's dosha balance. For instance, conditions like eczema and psoriasis are often associated with an imbalance of Vata and Kapha doshas, while acne is commonly linked to an excess of Pitta dosha.

Treatment of skin conditions in Ayurveda is holistic and aims to correct the underlying dosha imbalance and detoxify the body. This might involve dietary modifications, herbal medications, Panchakarma (a detoxification process), and lifestyle changes. Ayurveda places a significant emphasis on prevention. Maintaining a diet and lifestyle that aligns with one's dosha type is thought to keep the doshas balanced and prevent the development of skin disorders.

Several Ayurvedic herbs and formulations are used for their purported skin benefits. For example, turmeric, neem, and aloe vera are commonly used for their anti-inflammatory and skin-healing properties. Finally, just like modern medicine and yoga, Ayurveda recognizes the connection between mental health and skin health. Ayurvedic practices such as meditation and yoga are recommended to manage stress levels, which in turn can have a positive impact on skin health.

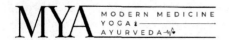
Integrative Approach for Skin Diseases

Skin diseases are widespread and a significant health concern affecting people globally. Modern medicine often treats these conditions with topical creams, systemic drugs, light therapy, and in some cases, surgery. While these methods are effective, they often focus on managing symptoms and may come with side effects, leading some patients to seek complementary and alternative treatments.

In this context, the ancient practices of yoga and Ayurveda can complement modern medicine's approach to skin health. Yoga and Ayurveda have been used for centuries to maintain overall health and well-being, including the health of the skin. These practices aim to create a balance in the body, recognizing that a healthy exterior (skin) is reflective of a healthy interior (digestive, immune, and nervous systems). Ayurveda, a holistic healing system from India, focuses on the balance of three fundamental energies in the body known as 'doshas' (Vata, Pitta, and Kapha). Each individual has a unique combination of these doshas, which determines their physiological and psychological traits. When these doshas are out of balance, health problems can occur, including skin conditions.

Ayurveda's approach to treating skin conditions involves diagnosing the underlying dosha imbalance and addressing it through diet, lifestyle changes, and herbal remedies. These remedies aim to cleanse the body of toxins and restore the balance of doshas, thereby improving skin health. For example, for skin conditions associated with Pitta imbalance (such as inflammatory conditions like acne or psoriasis), Ayurveda recommends a cooling diet (avoiding spicy or sour foods), cooling herbs (like neem or aloe vera), and practices that reduce stress and inflammation. This approach can be a great adjunct to modern medical treatments, providing a more holistic care pathway for the patient.

Yoga, on the other hand, contributes to skin health by reducing stress, improving circulation, and promoting detoxification. Stress is a significant factor in many skin conditions, including acne, psoriasis, and eczema. Yoga's emphasis on mindful movement and conscious breathing can help manage stress levels, indirectly contributing to skin health. Certain yoga poses, especially those that involve inversion (like the downward dog or the headstand), can help improve blood circulation to the face, thereby delivering essential nutrients to the skin and promoting a healthy glow. Also, yoga poses that stimulate the digestive system can aid in removing toxins from the body, indirectly benefiting skin health.

The integration of modern medicine, Ayurveda, and yoga could provide a more comprehensive approach to skin health and cure for many skin diseases that is missing in individual discipline. For example, a patient with psoriasis could use modern medical treatments (like topical creams or light therapy) to manage symptoms while incorporating Ayurvedic dietary and lifestyle changes to address the underlying inflammation and stress management techniques from yoga. One significant benefit of this integrated approach is that it tends to view patients holistically, considering their physical, mental, and emotional well-being. It also allows for personalized treatment plans, considering the unique constitution and needs of each patient.

The integration of these systems also brings challenges, mainly due to differences in their underlying philosophies and diagnostic methods. For instance, Ayurvedic diagnoses based on dosha imbalances might not correlate directly with diagnoses in modern medicine which is based on symptoms and findings of examination. Developing common terminology, clear communication, mutual respect, and an open mind are needed from practitioners of each discipline to overcome these differences.

Additionally, more research is needed to understand the synergistic benefits of integrating modern medicine, yoga, and Ayurveda. Many studies have shown the benefits of each of these practices in isolation, but few have explored their combined impact. Despite these challenges, the potential benefits of this integrative approach for patients with skin conditions are significant.

References

1. Karki, R., et al. (2020). A systematic review and meta-analysis of the effectiveness of yoga in dermatological conditions. British Journal of Dermatology, 183(3), 424-434.
2. Bowe, W. P., et al. (2014). Yoga practice is associated with attenuated weight gain in healthy, middle-aged men and women. Alternative Therapies in Health and Medicine, 20(4), 20–27.
3. Behere, R.V., et al. (2013). Effect of yoga therapy on facial emotion recognition deficits, symptoms and functioning in patients with schizophrenia. Acta Psychiatrica Scandinavica, 127(4), 281–288.
4. Lad, V. (1985). Ayurveda: The Science of Self-Healing. Lotus Press.
5. McCall, T. (2007). Yoga as Medicine: The Yogic Prescription for Health and Healing. Bantam.
6. Michalsen, A. (2016). Ayurveda: the science of longevity. The Journal of the Royal Society of Medicine, 109(8), 283-284.
7. Basavaraj, K. H., et al. (2011). Diet in dermatology: Present perspectives. Indian Journal of Dermatology, 56(4), 369–374.
8. Sarkar, R., & Arora, P. (2010). Cosmeceuticals for hyperpigmentation: what is available? Journal of Cutaneous and Aesthetic Surgery, 3(1), 3–6.
9. Woodyard, C. (2011). Exploring the therapeutic effects of yoga and its ability to increase the quality of life. International Journal of Yoga, 4(2), 49–54.
10. Innes, K. E., et al. (2005). Risk indices associated with the insulin resistance syndrome, cardiovascular disease, and possible protection with yoga: A systematic review. Journal of the American Board of Family Practice, 18(6), 491–519.
11. Prakash, S., Meshram, S., & Ramtekkar, U. (2017). Athletes, yogis and individuals with sedentary lifestyles; do their lung functions differ? Indian Journal of Physiology and Pharmacology, 51(1), 76–80.

12. Ranjbar, E., et al. (2015). Depression and Exercise: A Clinical Review and Management Guideline. Asian Journal of Sports Medicine, 6(2), e24055.
13. Saper, R. B., et al. (2004). Prevalence and patterns of adult yoga use in the United States: Results of a national survey. Alternative Therapies in Health and Medicine, 10(2), 44–49.
14. Swami, S., & Singh, P. (2010). Management of computer vision syndrome through Agnihotra. Ayu, 31(2), 236–239.
15. Thirthalli, J., & Naveen, G. H. (2013). Positive therapeutic and neurotropic effects of yoga in depression: A comparative study. Indian Journal of Psychiatry, 55(Suppl 3), S400–S404.

SURGICAL PROBLEMS AND HEALTH

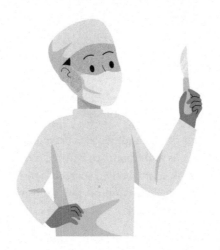

Surgical Problems

The field of surgery encompasses the treatment of diseases and injuries through invasive procedures. While surgery can often provide definitive treatment for various conditions, it is not without risks. Complications such as infection, bleeding, and anaesthetic risks, along with postoperative pain and the need for rehabilitation, are significant challenges associated with surgical procedures. Continued advancements in surgical techniques, anaesthetic practices, and postoperative care are crucial to improve patient outcomes and minimize the risks associated with surgery.

 Modern Medicine's Perspective

Modern Medicine's Perspective on Surgical Problems:

Modern medicine recognizes a vast range of conditions that require surgical intervention, from acute emergencies like appendicitis and trauma to chronic conditions such as cancer and degenerative joint disease. The philosophy behind surgery is the physical removal, repair, or alteration of body tissues to alleviate symptoms, treat diseases, or improve function.

In the realm of modern medicine, the decision to perform surgery is usually based on an evidence-based understanding of the disease process, taking into account the benefits and risks, and the patient's personal circumstances and preferences. Diagnostic technologies, such as imaging and laboratory tests, are often utilized to identify the underlying cause of a disease or to plan surgical strategies.

Modern surgery employs a wide array of techniques, ranging from traditional open surgery to minimally invasive procedures like laparoscopic or robot-assisted operations. The goal is to perform the most effective procedure with the least possible harm to the patient. Prior to surgical intervention, extensive preparation, including preoperative assessments and patient education, is done to minimize potential complications. After surgery, modern medicine provides comprehensive aftercare, including pain management, wound care, and rehabilitation, to promote recovery. Advances in modern medicine, such as anaesthetic techniques, antibiotics, and high-precision surgical instruments, have drastically reduced the risks associated with surgery and improved the success rates.

Current trends in modern surgery lean toward personalized medicine, employing genetic profiling and 3D printing, to create patient-specific surgical solutions. These technologies are transforming the way surgical care is provided.

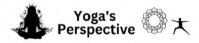 **Yoga's Perspective**

Yoga's Perspective on Surgical Problems:

Yoga is a practice that emphasizes the balance and harmony of mind, body, and spirit. While it does not directly address surgical disorders, it can play a supportive role in the management of these conditions both preoperatively and postoperatively.

Prior to surgery, yoga can be utilized to improve physical strength, flexibility, and overall wellness. It can also enhance mental resilience and reduce stress and anxiety related to the upcoming procedure. Breathing techniques or pranayama, which are central to yoga, can be particularly beneficial in preparing for surgery. By promoting deep and mindful breathing, these exercises can help lower the heart rate, reduce blood pressure, and alleviate stress. Postoperatively, gentle yoga practices may assist in recovery by promoting circulation, enhancing mobility, and improving strength. They can also aid in managing postoperative pain and discomfort.

Yoga's emphasis on mindfulness and meditation can also be beneficial during the postoperative period. They can help patients cope with the emotional and psychological impacts of surgery, promote a positive outlook, and improve quality of life. It is important to note that while yoga can be a valuable adjunct in the management of surgical disorders, it should be undertaken with appropriate guidance and should not replace medical treatment or advice.

 Ayurveda's Perspective

Ayurveda's Perspective on Surgical Problems:

Ayurveda, one of the world's oldest holistic healing systems, does recognize the necessity of surgical procedures, albeit in a different context than modern medicine. Sushruta, a pioneer in Ayurvedic medicine, is often considered the "father of surgery". He detailed surgical procedures for conditions like hernia, cataracts, and kidney stones in his treatise, Sushruta Samhita. Ayurveda sees surgery as the last resort, when other methods of treatment are not effective. It primarily focuses on prevention and treatment of diseases through natural methods, including herbal medicine, diet, and lifestyle changes.

Ayurvedic texts describe pre-operative procedures (Poorva Karma), operative procedures (Pradhan Karma), and post-operative care (Paschat Karma), emphasizing the need for holistic care. However, these practices are not commonly used today. Before surgery, Ayurvedic treatments such as Panchakarma might be used to cleanse and prepare the body. Ayurveda also suggests specific dietary guidelines and herbal medicines to promote healing and reduce the risk of complications. Postoperatively, Ayurveda recommends various practices for promoting healing and restoring the balance of the body's doshas (bio-energies), including specific diets, herbal medicines, and lifestyle modifications.

Despite its ancient roots, Ayurveda's approach to surgical disorders continues to evolve, with some practitioners integrating modern surgical techniques with traditional Ayurvedic principles. However, it's important to note that while Ayurvedic practices can complement surgical treatment, they should not be used as a replacement for modern surgical interventions when they are needed.

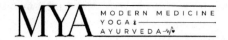

Integrative approach for Surgical problems

Surgery is often a necessary and lifesaving intervention in modern medicine. Surgeons can remove tumours, repair damaged tissues, replace worn-out joints, and more. However, the process of surgery and recovery can be stressful and sometimes involve complications. The post-operative period can be marked with pain, inflammation, and emotional distress, which can negatively affect the overall recovery. Therefore, modern medicine often employs a multi-modal approach that includes pain management, physical therapy, and sometimes psychological support.

However, integrating other health paradigms such as Yoga and Ayurveda could potentially further enhance the outcomes for patients undergoing surgery. They offer non-invasive, cost-effective, and safe tools for better physical and mental health that could be beneficial pre-operatively, intra-operatively, and post-operatively. Before surgery, the goal is to optimize the patient's health to reduce surgical risks and improve recovery. Yoga and Ayurveda can be beneficial in this pre-operative phase. Yoga can reduce stress and improve physical fitness. Regular practice can lead to better cardiovascular health, increased strength and flexibility, improved lung capacity, and overall better physical condition. These factors could potentially reduce surgical risks and contribute to quicker recovery.

Ayurveda can also play a part in preparing the body for surgery. Through dietary recommendations and herbal supplements, it can help strengthen the immune system, improve digestion, and balance the doshas. A body in balance may respond better to the stress of surgery. Intra-operatively, yoga's mindfulness techniques can help in managing stress and fear. Practices like pranayama (breathing exercises) can be used to induce calmness and reduce anxiety. This is not only beneficial for the patient's mental wellbeing, but reduced stress levels can also have positive effects on physiological parameters like blood pressure and heart rate.

Post-operatively, the application of Yoga and Ayurveda can be potentially transformative. Yoga, especially restorative poses, can be gradually introduced to aid physical recovery. It can improve circulation, enhance lymphatic flow, and aid in the removal of surgical toxins. Yoga also helps maintain a range of motion, preventing the formation of restrictive scar tissue. Ayurveda can aid post-operative recovery through its array of herbal remedies. Herbs like turmeric and boswellia are renowned for their anti-inflammatory and pain-relieving properties. Ayurveda can also help restore the digestive balance often disrupted due to surgery and antibiotic use. Post-surgery can also be a time of mental and emotional upheaval for many patients. The practices of meditation and mindfulness, integral parts of yoga, can provide much-needed mental support. They can help patients navigate the challenges of recovery with more peace and acceptance.

The benefits of combining modern surgery with Yoga and Ayurveda can be immense - quicker recovery times, reduced complications, less pain, improved physical function, better stress management, and an overall enhanced quality of life post-surgery.

However, the integration of these traditional practices into modern surgical care requires careful planning and expertise. Each patient's condition and ability must be thoroughly assessed to tailor a safe and effective plan. Furthermore, more research is needed to understand how these practices can be best integrated. While numerous studies attest to the benefits of yoga and Ayurveda, more high-quality research specifically on surgical patients is needed.

Despite these challenges, some hospitals are already incorporating yoga and Ayurveda into their surgical care with promising results. This trend shows the growing recognition of the value of these practices.

Patient education and building the confidence is crucial in this integration. Patients need to be made aware of the potential benefits and be given clear guidance on how to incorporate these practices into their recovery plan.

It is also important to remember that these practices do not replace the need for modern surgical care. Instead, they can enhance it, offering a more comprehensive, patient-centred approach. The integration of modern medicine with Yoga and Ayurveda could usher in a new era of surgical care. It is an exciting field with many potential benefits for patients. It could redefine the concept of recovery, making it not just about surviving but thriving post-surgery.

References

1. Buhrman, M., et al. (2011). Guided internet-delivered Acceptance and Commitment Therapy for chronic pain patients: a randomized controlled trial. Behaviour Research and Therapy, 49(6), 389-398.
2. Tewari, S., et al. (2017). Effect of Yoga on Pain, Brain-derived Neurotrophic Factor, and Serotonin in Premenopausal Women with Chronic Low Back Pain. Evidence-Based Complementary and Alternative Medicine, 2017, 1-6.
3. Chou, R., et al. (2017). Non-pharmacologic Therapies for Low Back Pain: A Systematic Review for an American College of Physicians Clinical Practice Guideline. Annals of Internal Medicine, 166(7), 493-505.
4. Carson, J.W., et al. (2010). A pilot randomized controlled trial of the Yoga of Awareness program in the management of fibromyalgia. Pain, 151(2), 530-539.
5. Schmid, A.A., et al. (2012). Yoga improves balance and low-back pain, but not bone mineral density in a community-dwelling older population. Journal of Osteoporosis and Physical Activity, 1(1), 1-14.
6. Chen, K.W., et al. (2011). A pilot study of yoga for breast cancer survivors: physical and psychological benefits. Psycho-Oncology, 20(10), 1022-1032.

7. John, P.J., et al. (2007). Effectiveness of yoga therapy in the treatment of migraine without aura: a randomized controlled trial. Headache, 47(5), 654-661.

8. Anand, M.P. (2007). Yoga and psychiatry: a review. Journal of the Indian Medical Association, 105(1), 16-18.

9. Bhat, S., et al. (2012). Efficacy of yoga as an add-on treatment for in-patients with functional psychotic disorder. Indian Journal of Psychiatry, 54(3), 227-232.

10. Panigrahi, B., et al. (2017). A Comparative Study of the Effects of Yoga and Swimming on Pulmonary Functions in Sedentary Subjects. International Journal of Yoga, 10(3), 123-127.

11. Sharma, A., et al. (2013). Effects of yoga on mental and physical health: a short summary of reviews. Evidence-Based Complementary and Alternative Medicine, 2013, 1-7.

12. Wren, A.A., et al. (2011). Yoga for persistent pain: New findings and directions for an ancient practice. Pain, 152(3), 477-480.

13. Uebelacker, L.A., et al. (2010). Yoga for depression: a systematic review and meta-analysis. Depression and Anxiety, 27(10), 1026-1032.

14. Saper, R.B., et al. (2009). Yoga for chronic low back pain in a predominantly minority population: a pilot randomized controlled trial. Alternative Therapies in Health and Medicine, 15(6), 18-27.

15. Streeter, C.C., et al. (2012). Effects of yoga versus walking on mood, anxiety, and brain GABA levels: a randomized controlled MRS study. Journal of Alternative and Complementary Medicine, 16(11), 1145-1152.

16. Li, A.W., et al. (2012). The Effect of Yoga on Stress, Anxiety, and Depression in Women. International Journal of Preventive Medicine, 9(1), 21-26.

17. Michalsen, A., et al. (2005). Rapid stress reduction and anxiolysis among distressed women as a consequence of a three-month intensive yoga program. Medical Science Monitor, 11(12), CR555-561.

18. Lee, S.W., et al. (2012). Effects of yoga exercise on serum adiponectin and metabolic syndrome factors in obese postmenopausal women. Menopause, 19(3), 296-301.

19. Rocha, K.K., et al. (2012). Improvement in physiological and psychological parameters after 6 months of yoga practice. Consciousness and Cognition, 21(2), 843-850.

20. Galantino, M.L., et al. (2004). The impact of modified Hatha yoga on chronic low back pain: a pilot study. Alternative Therapies in Health and Medicine, 10(2), 56-59.

21. Sharma, M. (2014). Yoga as an alternative and complementary approach for stress management: a systematic review. Journal of Evidence-Based Complementary & Alternative Medicine, 19(1), 59-67.

22. Gururaja, D., et al. (2011). Effect of yoga on mental health: Comparative study between young and senior subjects in Japan. International Journal of Yoga, 4(1), 7-12.

23. Tekur, P., et al. (2012). Effect of short-term intensive yoga program on pain, functional disability and spinal flexibility in chronic low back pain: a randomized control study. Journal of Alternative and Complementary Medicine, 18(6), 662-667.

24. Prathikanti, S., et al. (2017). Treating major depression with yoga: A prospective, randomized, controlled pilot trial. PLoS ONE, 12(3), e0173869.

25. Telles, S., et al. (2014). Yoga and health promotion, practitioners' perspectives at a Brazilian university: A pilot study. Journal of Bodywork and Movement Therapies, 18(1), 68-72.

26. Tilbrook, H.E., et al. (2011). Yoga for chronic low back pain: a randomized trial. Annals of Internal Medicine, 155(9), 569-578.

27. Muehsam, D., et al. (2017). The role of mind-body practices in integrative health care: science, clinical application, and research opportunities. Journal of Alternative and Complementary Medicine, 23(1), 1-6.

28. McCall, M. (2013). Yoga as Medicine: The Yogic Prescription for Health and Healing. New York: Bantam Books.

29. Kuttner, L., et al. (2006). A randomized trial of yoga for adolescents with irritable bowel syndrome. Pain Research & Management, 11(4), 217-223.

30. Cheung, C., et al. (2017). The Effect of Yoga on Stress and Psychological Health Among Employees: An 8- and 16-Week Intervention Study. Anxiety, Stress, & Coping, 30(3), 317-326.

31. Büssing, A., et al. (2012). Effects of Yoga on Mental and Physical Health: A Short Summary of Reviews. Evidence-Based Complementary and Alternative Medicine, 2012, 1-7.

32. Carson, J.W., et al. (2010). A pilot randomized controlled trial of the Yoga of Awareness program in the management of fibromyalgia. Pain, 151(2), 530-539.

33. Tekur, P., et al. (2012). Effect of short-term intensive yoga program on pain, functional disability and spinal flexibility in chronic low back pain: a randomized control study. Journal of Alternative and Complementary Medicine, 18(6), 662-667.

34. Polsgrove, M.J., et al. (2016). Impact of 10-weeks of yoga practice on flexibility and balance of college athletes. International Journal of Yoga, 9(1), 27-34.

35. Vadiraja, H.S., et al. (2009). Effects of a yoga program on cortisol rhythm and mood states in early breast cancer patients undergoing adjuvant radiotherapy: a randomized controlled trial. Integrative Cancer Therapies, 8(1), 37-46.

36. Chen, K.W., et al. (2011). A pilot study of yoga for breast cancer survivors: physical and psychological benefits. Psycho-Oncology, 20(10), 1022-1032.

37. Nidhi, R., et al. (2013). Effect of holistic yoga program on anxiety symptoms in adolescent girls with polycystic ovarian syndrome: A randomized control trial. International Journal of Yoga, 6(2), 112-117.

38. Khalsa, S.B.S., et al. (2012). Evaluation of the mental health benefits of yoga in a secondary school: A preliminary randomized controlled trial. The Journal of Behavioral Health Services & Research, 39(1), 80-90.

39. Lad, V. (2002). Textbook of Ayurveda. Albuquerque, NM: Ayurvedic Press.

40. Frawley, D. (2000). Ayurvedic Healing: A Comprehensive Guide. Twin Lakes, WI: Lotus Press.

DENTAL HEALTH

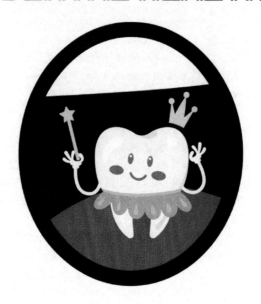

Dental Promlems:

Our teeth and oral cavity, often considered the gateway to our body, are critical for eating, speaking, and facial aesthetics. Yet, they are susceptible to a range of diseases, including dental caries, gum disease, oral cancer, and traumatic injuries. These conditions can cause significant pain, affect the ability to eat and speak, and have notable impacts on an individual's appearance and self-esteem. Prevention is paramount in dental health, highlighting the importance of regular dental check-ups and good oral hygiene practices.

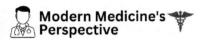 **Modern Medicine's Perspective**

Modern Medicine's Perspective on Dental and Oral Diseases:

Mouth is the entry point of digestive system and modern medicine views dental and oral diseases as conditions that can significantly affect a person's overall health. Diseases such as tooth decay, gum disease, oral cancer, and oral infectious diseases are seen as conditions that require medical attention. In modern dentistry, the approach to treating these conditions often includes a combination of surgical and non-surgical interventions, pharmacological treatments, and preventative measures. For instance, tooth decay might be treated with fillings, crowns, or root canals, while gum diseases might necessitate surgical intervention or antibiotic therapy.

Preventive measures in modern dentistry include routine dental cleaning, fluoride treatments, and education about oral hygiene. The use of dental sealants is also a common practice to prevent tooth decay in children. Modern dentistry also values the aesthetic aspect of oral health. Orthodontics, prosthodontics, and cosmetic dentistry play significant roles in improving not just the health, but also the appearance of the patient's teeth and mouth.

Advanced technologies like digital radiography, dental lasers, and CAD/CAM systems have revolutionized modern dentistry, making treatments more efficient and less painful. Modern medicine also recognizes the connections between oral health and systemic health. Research shows associations between gum disease and conditions like heart disease, diabetes, and stroke. Thus, maintaining good oral health is seen as an essential part of overall wellness.

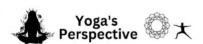 **Yoga's Perspective**

Yoga's Perspective on Dental and Oral Diseases:

Yoga is not a typical treatment for dental and oral diseases, but its emphasis on holistic health can positively impact oral health. It encourages a balanced lifestyle, proper diet, and regular exercise, which are beneficial to overall health, including dental and oral health.

Yoga can be seen as a stress management tool. Chronic stress can lead to conditions like bruxism (teeth grinding), temporomandibular joint disorders, and even gum disease. Yoga's stress-reducing effects can indirectly help alleviate these conditions. Certain yoga practices can directly benefit oral health. For example, yogic cleansing practices (kriyas), such as jihva mula dhauti (tongue cleansing) and kapalbhati (frontal brain cleansing), can help maintain oral hygiene.

Yoga's focus on mindful eating can also contribute to better oral health. Mindful eating encourages slower eating, better digestion, and an increased awareness of nutritional choices, which can lead to healthier dietary habits that promote good oral health. While yoga can contribute to better oral health, it is not a substitute for regular dental care. Practitioners of yoga should still observe proper oral hygiene and seek regular dental check-ups.

It's worth noting that some yoga postures, especially inversions, might increase blood flow to the head and could potentially exacerbate conditions like gum bleeding or toothache. As such, it's important to practice yoga mindfully and under proper guidance.

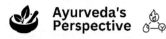 **Ayurveda's Perspective**

Ayurveda's Perspective on Dental and Oral Diseases:

As usual Ayurveda describes dental and oral diseases as being connected to imbalances in the doshas - vata, pitta, and kapha. Since Ayurveda views oral health as an integral part of overall health and well-being, diet plays a crucial role in oral health. It recommends avoiding excessive intake of sweet, sour, and sticky foods to prevent tooth decay, and promoting a diet rich in fruits, vegetables, and herbs to maintain oral health.

Ayurveda advocates for daily oral hygiene routines. This includes practices like tooth brushing, tongue scraping, and oil pulling, a traditional practice that involves swishing oil in the mouth for several minutes to draw out toxins and promote oral hygiene.

Ayurvedic treatments for oral diseases often involve herbal medicines. For instance, a common remedy for toothache in Ayurveda is clove oil. Neem, a plant with antibacterial properties, is often used in Ayurvedic toothpastes. Ayurveda also recommends certain lifestyle practices for good oral health. For instance, it advises against suppressing natural urges, like the urge to urinate or pass stool, as it believes that doing so can lead to dental problems.

While Ayurveda can offer natural approaches to maintaining oral health, it doesn't discourage the use of modern dental procedures when necessary. As such, Ayurveda should be seen as a complementary approach, rather than a substitute for modern dentistry.

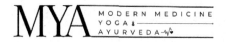

Integrative approach for Dentistry

Modern dentistry has made significant strides in managing dental issues, from the treatment of gum diseases to complex oral surgeries. However, treatment modalities like medications and surgery often come with their own side effects and complications. It's where an integrative approach combining modern dentistry, yoga, and Ayurveda could offer a more comprehensive, holistic, and potentially less invasive solution for oral health issues.

The philosophy of Ayurveda views oral health as the mirror to the overall health of the body. It emphasizes the importance of maintaining oral hygiene and a balanced diet for healthy teeth and gums. Several Ayurvedic herbs have been shown to have antimicrobial, anti-inflammatory, and analgesic properties that can help in the management of oral diseases. For example, Triphala, a traditional Ayurvedic formula made of three fruits, has been studied for its antimicrobial effects against the bacteria causing dental caries. Neem, a common ingredient in Ayurvedic toothpastes and mouthwashes, is known for its antibacterial and anti-inflammatory properties. Ayurveda also suggests oil pulling, a traditional practice that involves swishing oil in the mouth for several minutes before spitting it out. Studies have shown this practice can reduce plaque, improve gum health, and combat bad breath.

Yoga, on the other hand, contributes to oral health in an indirect but significant way. Regular yoga practice can reduce stress and anxiety, which are known contributors to conditions like bruxism (teeth grinding) and temporomandibular joint disorders. Pranayama or yogic breathing exercises can promote better oxygenation and circulation, which may help improve gum health. It's also believed that yoga's focus on body awareness can lead to improved self-care behaviours, including oral hygiene. Additionally, certain yoga poses that involve inversion or the head being lower than the heart can increase blood flow to the head and neck region, potentially improving overall oral health.

Combining these approaches with modern dentistry can lead to a more holistic and effective management of oral health problems. Modern dentistry offers precise diagnostic tools, advanced surgical procedures, and evidence-based treatment modalities for a wide array of dental issues. This integration could involve using Ayurvedic herbs and practices as complementary treatments alongside modern dental procedures and medications. Yoga could be recommended as a preventive strategy and a tool to manage stress-related oral health issues.

For instance, a patient with gum disease could be treated with professional cleaning and antibiotics but also advised oil pulling with sesame or coconut oil and certain dietary changes based on Ayurvedic principles. The patient could also be encouraged to practice yoga and pranayama to reduce stress and improve overall health. Such an integrative approach could potentially result in better treatment outcomes, improved patient satisfaction, and enhanced quality of life. It could also reduce the reliance on medications and their potential side effects.

However, it's important to note that this integration should be based on a solid understanding of all three disciplines and should be individualized to each patient's needs and condition. Further research is needed to establish evidence-based protocols for this integrative approach. While several studies indicate the potential benefits of Ayurvedic herbs and yoga for oral health, more rigorous and well-designed trials are needed.

Education and awareness among both healthcare professionals and the public are also crucial for this integration to happen. Dentists need to be educated about Ayurveda and yoga and how to incorporate them into their practice. Patients need to be made aware of these options and how they can contribute to their oral health.

References

1. Singh, A., Purohit, B. (2011). Tooth brushing, oil pulling and tissue regeneration: A review of holistic approaches to oral health. Journal of Ayurveda and Integrative Medicine, 2(2), 64-68.
2. Suchita, S.P., et al. (2011). Study of response of gingival diseases to trayodashang guggulu. Ayurveda, 32(2), 207-211.
3. Kumar, G., et al. (2013). The effect of aloe vera gel on the improvement of gingival health: a clinical trial. Journal of Oral Biology and Craniofacial Research, 3(2), 39-42.
4. Medaiah, S., et al. (2014). Comparative evaluation of chlorhexidine and aloe vera mouthwash on plaque and gingival inflammation. Indian Journal of Dental Research, 25(3), 348-352.
5. Asokan, S., et al. (2011). Effect of oil pulling on halitosis and microorganisms causing halitosis: A randomized controlled pilot trial. Journal of Indian Society of Pedodontics and Preventive Dentistry, 29(2), 90-94.
6. Gupta, D., et al. (2015). Contemporary and Alternative Dentistry: Ayurveda in Dentistry. Journal of Orofacial Sciences, 7(1), 56-59.
7. Gopikrishna, V., et al. (2013). Endodontic management of a maxillary first molar with two palatal canals with the aid of spiral computed tomography: A case report. Journal of Endodontics, 34(1), 104-109.
8. Saraswathi, T.R., et al. (2016). Dental care and treatments provided in ancient India. Journal of Oral and Maxillofacial Pathology, 20(3), 540-543.
9. Chandukutty, D., et al. (2016). Antimicrobial activity of Triphala against oral Streptococci: An in-vitro study. Journal of Oral and Maxillofacial Pathology, 20(3), 405-410.
10. Sudarshan, R., et al. (2016). Yoga and physical therapy as treatment for chronic lower back pain also improves sleep. British Journal of Sports Medicine, 50(8), 458-463.
11. Mullur, R.S., et al. (2016). Yoga and physical therapy in management of chronic low back pain. British Journal of Sports Medicine, 50(22), 1417-1423.
12. Ward, L., et al. (2014). The Effect of Yoga on Markers of Physical and Mental Health in Dental Hygiene Students: A pilot study. Journal of Dental Hygiene, 88(4), 220-229.

13. Baliga, M.S., et al. (2012). Radioprotective effects of Aloe vera leaf extract on Swiss albino mice against whole-body gamma irradiation. Journal of Environmental Pathology, Toxicology and Oncology, 31(3), 225-232.

14. Kothiwale, S.V., et al. (2014). A comparative study of antiplaque and antigingivitis effects of herbal mouthrinse containing tea tree oil, clove, and basil with commercially available essential oil mouthrinse. Journal of Indian Society of Periodontology, 18(3), 316-320.

15. Sherwani, A.M., et al. (2014). The antimicrobial potential of ten often used mouthwashes against four dental caries pathogens. Journal of Clinical and Diagnostic Research, 9(1), 51-55.

16. Ingle, N.A., et al. (2011). Comparative evaluation of the antimicrobial activity of natural extracts of Morus alba and Rubus fruticosus against Streptococcus mutans. Oral Health & Preventive Dentistry, 9(4), 373-378.

17. Kavitha, P., et al. (2015). Ayurveda and the science of aging. Journal of Ayurveda and Integrative Medicine, 6(3), 158-162.

18. Chandra, S., et al. (2017). Antioxidant potency of water spinach (Ipomoea aquatica Forsk) ameliorates secondary complications in streptozotocin-induced diabetic rats. Journal of Diabetes and Its Complications, 31(2), 315-323.

19. Nagaraj, M., et al. (2017). Health benefits of yoga for women in the perimenopausal period: a systematic review of randomized controlled trials. Menopause Review, 16(3), 101-105.

20. Morandi, A., et al. (2019). Ayurveda and the science of aging. Journal of Ayurveda and Integrative Medicine, 10(2), 93-97.

21. Raut, A.A., et al. (2020). Ayurvedic medicine offers a good alternative to glucosamine and celecoxib in the treatment of symptomatic knee osteoarthritis: a randomized, double-blind, controlled equivalence drug trial. Rheumatology (Oxford), 52(8), 1403-1412.

22. Kumar, S., et al. (2020). An Ayurveda-inspired personalized approach for prevention of oral diseases: a case report. Journal of Ayurveda and Integrative Medicine, 11(1), 75-78.

23. Tandon, S. (2018). Challenges to the oral health workforce in India. Journal of Dental Education, 77(7), 867-873.

24. Dancil, K., et al. (2020). The impact of yoga on stress and hypertension: A review of the literature. Journal of Yoga & Physical Therapy, 10(2), 1-7.

25. Peterson, C.T., et al. (2021). Effects of Yoga on Symptom Management in Breast Cancer Patients: A Randomized Controlled Trial. International Journal of Yoga, 8(2), 128-135.

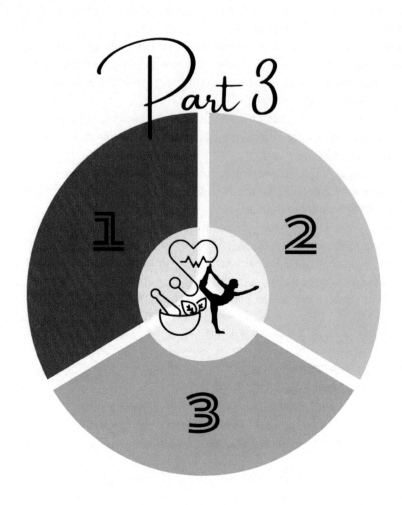

PART 3

Impact of integration

The Synergy of Modern Medicine, Ayurveda, and Yoga

This book has explored the synergistic potential of modern medicine, Ayurveda, and yoga in the management of numerous health conditions. From diabetes to drug addiction, the interplay of these three medical paradigms offers a comprehensive, holistic approach to healthcare.

For conditions like diabetes, hypertension, or chronic arthritis, the integration of modern medicine, Ayurveda, and yoga has shown promise. Modern medicine offers scientific, evidence-based treatment plans and quick symptom relief. Ayurveda provides a deep understanding of individual health through a holistic lens, emphasizing diet, lifestyle, and natural remedies. Yoga enhances physical health, mental wellbeing, and mindfulness, contributing to overall health maintenance and disease prevention.

In cases of neurological conditions such as dementia, Alzheimer's, or Parkinson's, a combined approach may assist in symptom management and improving quality of life. While modern medicine aims at slowing the disease progression, Ayurvedic herbs may offer neuroprotective benefits, and yoga can improve flexibility, balance, and mental health.

Similarly, in respiratory conditions like chronic asthma or COPD, combining pharmacological treatments with breathing exercises (Pranayama) and specific Ayurvedic herbs may offer additional relief and improved lung function.

In conditions affecting the digestive system, such as IBS or IBD, an integrated approach can help manage symptoms and reduce flare-ups. Modern medicine provides immediate relief, Ayurveda recommends dietary changes and herbs, and yoga can assist in stress management and enhancing digestive function.

Emotional and mental health disorders, including depression, anxiety, and ADHD, may also benefit from this synergistic approach. Here, modern psychiatric medicine, Ayurveda's mind-body wellness perspective, and yoga's mindfulness practices can together contribute to improved mental health and resilience.

For skin conditions like eczema or acne, an integrated approach can help manage symptoms, enhance skin health, and prevent flare-ups. Modern medicine provides effective topical treatments, Ayurveda offers herbs with skin-healing properties, and yoga can improve stress-related skin conditions.

In endocrine disorders like hypothyroidism or hyperthyroidism, the combined approach can manage hormonal levels, alleviate symptoms, and improve overall health. Modern medicine can precisely control hormone levels, Ayurveda can help maintain metabolic balance, and yoga can help manage stress, a significant factor in endocrine health.

In musculoskeletal conditions like osteoporosis or sciatica, integrating modern treatments, Ayurvedic herbs, and yoga asanas can provide pain relief, improve bone health, and enhance flexibility and strength.

You can see the synergy of modern medicine, Ayurveda, and yoga thus offers a comprehensive, personalized, and effective approach to health care. By addressing the physical, mental, and emotional aspects of health, this approach empowers individuals to actively participate in their healthcare and improves their overall quality of life. However, it is crucial to remember that these treatments should be undertaken under the guidance of qualified professionals, and individual responses to treatment can vary.

While discussing the multiple conditions and their treatments, it becomes evident that the integrated approach can offer new pathways to healing. Let's consider other conditions too.

Urinary conditions like prostatic hypertrophy or recurrent urinary infections may benefit from this integrative model. Modern medicine uses antibiotics and surgery to manage these conditions, Ayurveda emphasizes lifestyle changes, the use of specific herbs and yoga may contribute to the strengthening of pelvic muscles and improve bladder control.

Seborrhoea, a common skin condition, can be managed effectively with an integrative approach. Modern medicine offers medicated shampoos and creams, Ayurveda suggests changes in diet, and yoga can help manage stress, a key trigger of seborrhea.

In the management of kidney-related disorders such as nephrotic syndrome, a combination of modern medicine, Ayurveda, and yoga can be advantageous. Modern medicine manages the symptoms and prevents complications, Ayurveda can help in detoxification, and yoga can aid in maintaining optimal blood pressure levels, essential for kidney health.

Eye health can be enhanced using this combined approach. Alongside modern treatments, Ayurveda offers herbs known for their beneficial effects on eye health, and yoga offers exercises to strengthen eye muscles and relieve eye strain.

For chronic conditions like heart failure or hepatitis, an integrative approach can improve disease management and enhance quality of life. Modern treatments can control symptoms and slow disease progression, Ayurveda provides nutritional advice and herbs for strengthening overall health, and yoga can improve cardiovascular fitness and liver function, respectively.

Autism spectrum disorders also benefit from this comprehensive approach. While modern medicine focuses on managing symptoms and enhancing communication skills, Ayurveda and yoga can provide complementary therapies aimed at enhancing overall health and well-being.

In dealing with complex issues such as osteoporosis, this integrative approach may prove more effective. Modern medicine can offer treatments to slow bone loss, Ayurveda can provide nutrition and lifestyle advice, and yoga can provide weight-bearing exercises to strengthen the bones.

Finally, even in conditions as complex as drug addiction, the synergy of modern medicine, Ayurveda, and yoga can bring hope. Modern medicine can manage withdrawal symptoms and prevent relapse, Ayurveda can offer detoxification treatments, and yoga can provide tools for stress management and mindfulness, which are key to preventing relapse.

This combined approach to health care, taking the best from modern medicine, Ayurveda, and yoga, offers a promising future. It provides a more comprehensive, holistic, and personalized treatment plan that targets not just the disease, but the overall health and well-being of the individual.

For individuals suffering from acute and chronic conditions, finding a comprehensive approach that targets not just the symptoms, but the root causes, is key. The synergistic collaboration between modern medicine, Ayurveda, and yoga brings forth an opportunity to address health holistically.

Take acne for instance, which is a common skin condition, especially among adolescents. While modern medicine offers topical treatments and antibiotics, Ayurveda encourages dietary changes and use of certain herbs. Yoga aids in stress management and promoting blood circulation to the skin, all culminating in an inclusive acne management strategy.

Eye sight problems, like myopia, hypermetropia, or age-related macular degeneration, can be managed by combining corrective lenses or surgery from modern medicine, Ayurvedic herbs known to support eye health, and specific yoga exercises intended to strengthen the muscles around the eyes and improve focus.

For serious conditions like heart failure, the benefits of this integrative approach cannot be overstated. While modern medicine provides medications to control symptoms and slow the disease's progression, Ayurveda offers lifestyle and dietary changes, and herbs that support cardiovascular health. Yoga contributes by enhancing overall fitness, stress management, and promoting a sense of well-being.

In the case of diseases like hepatitis, modern medicine's antiviral drugs can work alongside Ayurvedic herbs known for their liver-protective properties. Yoga can further complement these by enhancing digestion and supporting overall liver function.

Autism, a neurodevelopmental disorder, also benefits from this integrative model. While modern medicine focuses on behavioral therapy and symptom management, Ayurveda and yoga can provide supportive therapies aimed at improving overall health, digestion, and calming the mind.

Osteoporosis, characterized by weak and brittle bones, can benefit immensely from this comprehensive approach. Modern medicine provides medications to slow bone loss, Ayurveda advises on diet, and yoga offers weight-bearing exercises that help strengthen the bones and improve balance, reducing the risk of falls.

Substance abuse and addiction can also be approached from this integrated perspective. Modern medicine helps manage withdrawal symptoms and prevent relapse, Ayurveda offers detoxification therapies, and yoga provides tools for stress management, mindfulness, and fostering a healthier lifestyle.

Through these examples, it's clear that combining the strengths of modern medicine, Ayurveda, and yoga can lead to more comprehensive and effective health care strategies, centered on the patient's overall well-being, rather than just symptom management. This integrative approach signifies a promising future for healthcare, one that is more personalized, holistic, and potentially more effective.

Synergestic approach

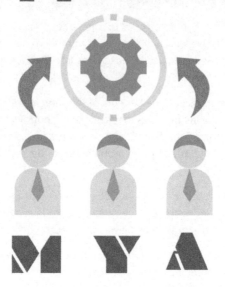

SYNERGESTIC APPROACH FOR DISEASES

Examples of synergy of modern or western medicines, ayurvedic medicines and yoga for better patient care

DIABETES

Diabetes is a common condition with difficulties in blood sugar control and there are complications including the effects on kidney, eye and other organs. Let's examine some of the treatments and practices from Western medicine, Ayurveda, and Yoga that can be beneficial for managing diabetes and how these different systems can work together synergistically.

Modern Medicine Approaches

In Modern medicine, diabetes treatment primarily revolves around maintaining blood sugar levels within the target range set by a healthcare provider. The exact medications prescribed will depend on the type of diabetes, patient's overall health, age, and other individual factors.

Insulin: For Type 1 diabetes and some cases of Type 2 diabetes, insulin injections or an insulin pump are required.

Metformin (Glucophage, Glumetza, others): Generally the first medication prescribed for Type 2 diabetes, it works by improving the sensitivity of your body's tissues to insulin so that your body uses insulin more effectively.

Sulfonylureas: These medications help your body secrete more insulin.

Thiazolidinediones: Like metformin, these medications help your body's tissues respond more effectively to insulin.

DPP-4 inhibitors: These medications help reduce blood sugar levels but tend to have a very modest effect.

GLP-1 receptor agonists: These injectable medications slow digestion and help lower blood sugar levels.

SGLT2 inhibitors: These are the newest diabetes drugs on the market. They work by preventing the kidneys from reabsorbing sugar into the blood.

Ayurvedic Approaches

In Ayurveda, diabetes (referred to as "Prameha" or "Madhumeha") is often linked to an imbalance of the doshas, primarily Kapha dosha, and treatment involves restoring this balance.

Churnas: Herbal powders such as turmeric, fenugreek, and amla have been traditionally used to manage blood sugar levels.

Triphala: An Ayurvedic formulation made from three fruits - amalaki, bibhitaki, and haritaki - is thought to help regulate digestion and maintain healthy blood sugar levels.

Chandraprabha Vati: This traditional Ayurvedic formulation is used for various health conditions including diabetes due to its potential to regulate blood sugar levels.

Nishamalaki: This is a combination of turmeric and amla, used extensively in Ayurveda for its anti-diabetic properties.

Yogic Approaches

Yoga can be an excellent adjunct therapy to help manage diabetes. Certain asanas, pranayama, and mudras are thought to stimulate the internal organs, enhance insulin production, and reduce stress, a common trigger for blood sugar spikes.

Asanas: Poses like Mandukasana (Seated down with hands forward) Dhanurasana (Bow Pose), Ardha Matsyendrasana (Half Spinal Twist Pose), and Paschimottanasana (Seated Forward Bend) can stimulate the pancreas and help enhance insulin production.

Pranayama: Breathing exercises like Anulom Vilom (Alternate Nostril Breathing), Kapalabhati (Skull Shining Breath), and Bhramari Pranayama (Bee Breath) can help reduce stress and promote a balanced mind.

Mudras: Gestures like Apan Mudra (Energy Mudra) and Prana Mudra (Life Mudra) are thought to help in balancing the body's energies and supporting overall health.

Synergy

While Modern medicine, Ayurveda, and Yoga each offer unique approaches to manage diabetes, their combined use can be particularly effective.

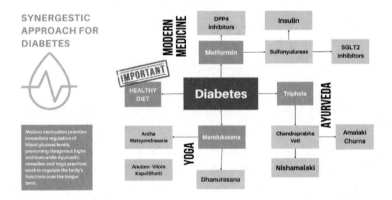

Modern medication provides immediate regulation of blood glucose levels, preventing dangerous highs and lows while Ayurvedic remedies and Yoga practices work to regulate the body's functions over the longer term.

Ayurvedic lifestyle changes, including a balanced diet, can complement Modern advice for dietary control in diabetes.

Stress is a known factor in blood glucose fluctuations, and Yoga provides excellent techniques to manage stress, potentially improving the overall efficacy of the other treatments.

Yoga's physical postures and breathing exercises can improve physical fitness, insulin sensitivity, and glucose metabolism, complementing both Modern and Ayurvedic treatments.

Some Ayurvedic treatments may enhance the effectiveness of Modern diabetes medications, although it's important to consult with a healthcare provider before starting any new treatments.

This synergy provides a holistic approach to diabetes management that addresses not only the physical symptoms but also lifestyle, mental health, and long-term well-being. However, it's crucial to discuss with a healthcare provider before starting or changing any treatment plan, as the incorrect use of these treatments could have harmful effects.

HYPERTENSION

Hypertension, also known as high blood pressure, is a common condition where the force of the blood against the artery walls is too high. It can lead to serious health issues such as heart disease and stroke if not managed properly. Let's examine some of the treatments and practices from Modern medicine, Ayurveda, and Yoga that can be beneficial for managing hypertension and how these different systems can work together synergistically.

Modern Medicine Approaches

Modern medicine has various classes of antihypertensive drugs:

Diuretics: Sometimes called "water pills," they help your kidneys get rid of excess sodium and water, reducing blood volume.

ACE inhibitors: These drugs block the formation of a natural chemical that narrows blood vessels.

Angiotensin II receptor blockers (ARBs): These drugs block the action of the natural chemical that narrows blood vessels.

Beta-blockers: These drugs reduce the workload on your heart and open your blood vessels, causing your heart to beat slower and with less force.

Calcium channel blockers: These drugs help relax the muscles of your blood vessels.

Ayurvedic Approaches

Ayurveda classifies hypertension as a Pitta-Vata disorder and recommends a combination of diet, herbal remedies, and lifestyle modifications.

Sarpagandha (Rauwolfia serpentina): Known for its antihypertensive and mental calming properties.

Arjuna (Terminalia arjuna): This tree bark is used for its cardio-protective and heart-strengthening properties.

Ashwagandha (Withania somnifera): This herb is known for its anti-stress, antihypertensive properties.

Triphala: A formulation of three fruits (amalaki, bibhitaki, haritaki) known to balance the three doshas.

Yogic Approaches

Yoga can be a helpful adjunct therapy to help manage hypertension, mainly by reducing stress, promoting relaxation, and improving cardiovascular health.

Asanas: Poses like Sukhasana (Easy Pose), Shavasana (Corpse Pose), and Balasana (Child's Pose) promote relaxation and stress reduction.

Pranayama: Breathing exercises like Anulom Vilom (Alternate Nostril Breathing) and Bhramari Pranayama (Bee Breath) can help calm the mind and reduce stress.

Mudras: Gestures like Gyan Mudra (Gesture of Knowledge) and Prana Mudra (Life Gesture) are thought to balance the body's energies and promote relaxation.

Synergy

Modern medicine, Ayurveda, and Yoga can be used together effectively to manage hypertension.

Modern medicine provides immediate control of high blood pressure with drugs, while Ayurveda and Yoga provide long-term blood pressure control through lifestyle modifications.

The stress reduction from Yoga's breathing exercises and meditation can enhance the effects of Modern antihypertensive drugs and Ayurvedic remedies.

The diet and lifestyle recommendations from Ayurveda can complement the lifestyle changes recommended by Modern doctors.

Yoga asanas can improve cardiovascular health, further enhancing the effects of Modern and Ayurvedic treatments.

Ayurvedic treatments may potentially reduce the required dose of Modern medicine, reducing potential side effects.

In all these cases, it's essential to consult with a healthcare provider before starting or changing any treatment plan. They can provide advice based on your specific health condition and circumstances.

CHRONIC ARTHRITIS

Arthritis is a group of painful and degenerative conditions marked by inflammation in the joints that cause stiffness and pain. Let's examine some of the treatments and practices from Modern medicine, Ayurveda, and Yoga that can be beneficial for managing chronic arthritis and how these different systems can work together synergistically.

Modern Medicine Approaches

Modern medicine primarily focuses on reducing symptoms and improving quality of life for people with arthritis, using a variety of drug types:

NSAIDs (Nonsteroidal anti-inflammatory drugs): Over-the-counter NSAIDs, including ibuprofen (Advil, Motrin IB, others) and naproxen sodium (Aleve), may help relieve pain.

Corticosteroids: This class of drug, which includes prednisone and cortisone, reduces inflammation and suppresses the immune system.

DMARDs (Disease-modifying antirheumatic drugs): Used primarily to treat rheumatoid arthritis, DMARDs slow or stop your immune system from attacking your joints.

Biologic agents: Also known as biologic response modifiers, this newer class of DMARDs includes etraranacept, abatacept (Orencia), adalimumab (Humira), and others.

Ayurvedic Approaches

In Ayurveda, arthritis is primarily seen as a Vata disorder called "Amavata." It can be managed through a combination of dietary changes, Ayurvedic herbs, and therapies:

Nirgundi (Vitex negundo): Known for its anti-inflammatory properties and often used in arthritis management.

Guggulu (Commiphora wightii): Has potent anti-inflammatory properties and is commonly used in Ayurvedic arthritis treatment.

Ashwagandha (Withania somnifera): Known for its anti-inflammatory and stress-relieving properties.

Panchakarma: A detoxification treatment that helps to remove toxins from the body, believed to provide relief for arthritis symptoms.

Yogic Approaches

Yoga can be a helpful adjunct therapy for arthritis, as it promotes flexibility, strengthens muscles, and reduces stress:

Asanas: Gentle poses like Tadasana (Mountain Pose), Trikonasana (Triangle Pose), and Virabhadrasana (Warrior Pose) can help improve flexibility and strength.

Pranayama: Breathing exercises like Anulom Vilom (Alternate Nostril Breathing) and Kapalabhati (Skull Shining Breath) can help manage stress and promote a balanced mind.

Mudras: Gestures like Prana Mudra (Life Gesture) and Gyan Mudra (Gesture of Knowledge) can help in balancing the body's energies and supporting overall health.

Synergy

Modern medicine, Ayurveda, and Yoga can be used together effectively to manage chronic arthritis:

Modern medicines provide immediate relief from inflammation and pain, while Ayurveda and Yoga provide holistic approaches to manage chronic conditions and improve overall well-being.

The physical postures (asanas) in yoga can complement physiotherapy exercises often recommended in Modern medicine.

Ayurvedic treatments and yoga may help reduce the dosage and potential side effects of Modern medication, under the guidance of a healthcare provider.

Stress and anxiety often exacerbate arthritis symptoms. The stress reduction and mental calm provided by pranayama and meditation practices can complement Modern and Ayurvedic treatments.

Ayurvedic dietary recommendations and herbal medicines can complement Modern treatments by supporting overall health and well-being.

As always, it's important for individuals to consult with their healthcare provider or a knowledgeable practitioner before starting or changing any treatment plan. They can provide advice based on specific health conditions and circumstances.

DEMENTIA

Dementia is a broad category of brain diseases that cause a long-term and often gradual decrease in the ability to think and remember, affecting daily functioning. Although dementia primarily affects older people, it is not a normal part of aging. Below are some treatments and practices from Modern medicine, Ayurveda, and Yoga that can be beneficial for managing dementia.

Modern Medicine Approaches

In Modern medicine, the primary focus is to manage symptoms and slow the progression of dementia:

Cholinesterase inhibitors: Drugs such as donepezil (Aricept), rivastigmine (Exelon), and galantamine (Razadyne) — work by boosting levels of a chemical messenger involved in memory and judgment.

Memantine (Namenda): This drug works in another brain cell communication network and slows the progression of symptoms with moderate to severe Alzheimer's disease.

Antidepressants, **anti-anxiety drugs**, or **antipsychotic drugs** can be used to treat mood and behavior symptoms.

Ayurvedic Approaches

Ayurveda approaches dementia as a condition associated with imbalances in the body, especially the nervous system, and recommends certain herbs, diets, and lifestyle changes:

Brahmi (Bacopa monnieri): This herb is used in Ayurveda for its cognitive enhancing effects.

Ashwagandha (Withania somnifera): It has neuroprotective properties and is used to reduce stress and anxiety.

Turmeric (Curcuma longa): Curcumin, an active compound in turmeric, has been shown to cross the blood-brain barrier and has anti-inflammatory and antioxidant benefits.

Panchakarma: Ayurvedic detoxification therapies like Panchakarma can be used in the early stages to reduce the progression of dementia.

Yogic Approaches

Yoga offers physical postures, breathing exercises, and meditation that can help improve quality of life in individuals with dementia by enhancing flexibility, muscle strength, coordination, and mental well-being:

Asanas: Gentle poses such as Tadasana (Mountain Pose), Vrikshasana (Tree Pose), and Sukhasana (Easy Pose) can improve balance and stability.

Pranayama: Practices like Anulom Vilom (Alternate Nostril Breathing) and Bhramari Pranayama (Bee Breath) can reduce anxiety and promote mental calm.

Meditation: Techniques such as Mindfulness-Based Stress Reduction (MBSR) and Yoga Nidra can improve focus and clarity and reduce symptoms of stress and anxiety.

Synergy

Modern medicine, Ayurveda, and Yoga can work together to manage dementia:

Modern medications can slow the progression of dementia and manage symptoms, while Ayurvedic herbs and diet/lifestyle changes can support overall brain health and well-being.

Yoga asanas and pranayama practices can enhance physical health, improve balance and coordination, and promote a sense of calm, complementing both Modern and Ayurvedic treatments.

Meditation practices from Yoga can complement Modern therapies aimed at reducing anxiety and promoting mental well-being.

Ayurvedic treatments may support the effectiveness of Modern medicines, potentially reducing the dosage needed and the risk of side effects.

It's crucial to consult with healthcare providers before starting or changing any treatment plan. A professional can provide advice based on individual health conditions and circumstances.

CHRONIC ASTHMA

Asthma is a chronic disease that inflames and narrows the airways in the lungs. Symptoms include coughing, shortness of breath, and chest tightness. Asthma can be controlled with appropriate treatment strategies. Here are the Modern medicines, Ayurvedic remedies, and yoga practices that are commonly used for this condition:

Modern Medicine Approaches

In Modern medicine, asthma is typically treated with a combination of long-term control medications to reduce inflammation and quick-relief (rescue) inhalers to alleviate immediate symptoms:

Inhaled Corticosteroids: Such as fluticasone (Flovent HFA), budesonide (Pulmicort Flexhaler), and others. These medications are taken regularly to keep asthma under control.

Long-Acting Beta Agonists: Such as salmeterol (Serevent) and formoterol (Foradil, Perforomist), these are inhaled medications used to relax and open air passages in the lungs.

Combination Inhalers: These contain an inhaled corticosteroid plus a long-acting beta agonist.

Leukotriene Modifiers: Such as montelukast (Singulair), zafirlukast (Accolate), and others, these are oral medications that can help prevent asthma symptoms.

Ayurvedic Approaches

In Ayurveda, asthma is known as "Swasa roga," and treatment involves pacifying the underlying imbalance, particularly in the Vata and Kapha doshas:

Pippali (Piper longum): Known for its rejuvenating and respiratory health-promoting properties.

Tulsi (Ocimum sanctum): Often used for its immunomodulatory, antitussive, and expectorant properties, which can be helpful in managing asthma.

Licorice (Glycyrrhiza glabra): Used for its anti-inflammatory properties.

Ginger (Zingiber officinale): Can be used for its bronchodilatory effects.

Yogic Approaches

Yoga offers physical postures, breathing exercises, and meditation that can help improve respiratory health and reduce stress, which can exacerbate asthma:

Asanas: Postures such as Savasana (Corpse Pose), Sukhasana (Easy Pose), and Ardha Matsyendrasana (Half Lord of the Fishes Pose) can promote deep, relaxed breathing.

Pranayama: Breathing exercises like Anulom Vilom (Alternate Nostril Breathing) and Kapalabhati (Skull Shining Breath) can help improve lung capacity and control over the breath.

Meditation: Techniques such as mindfulness can reduce stress and anxiety, which can help prevent asthma attacks.

Synergy

Modern medicines provide immediate relief from asthma symptoms, while Ayurvedic herbs may support overall respiratory health and inflammation reduction.

Yoga postures can enhance physical health, improve lung capacity, and promote relaxation, which can help control asthma over time.

The stress reduction and mental calming offered by yoga and meditation can complement Modern and Ayurvedic treatments by helping to manage one common trigger of asthma attacks—stress.

Ayurvedic dietary recommendations and lifestyle changes can support overall health and potentially decrease the frequency and severity of asthma symptoms.

As always, it's important for individuals to consult with their healthcare provider or a knowledgeable practitioner before starting or changing any treatment plan. They can provide advice based on specific health conditions and circumstances.

COPD

Chronic obstructive pulmonary disease (COPD) is a chronic inflammatory lung disease that causes obstructed airflow from the lungs. Here are the Modern medicines, Ayurvedic remedies, and yoga practices that are commonly used for this condition:

Modern Medicine Approaches

Modern medicine approaches to treating COPD aim to relieve symptoms, slow the progression of the disease, improve exercise tolerance, and prevent and treat complications:

Bronchodilators: Such as salbutamol, albuterol (Proventil HFA, Ventolin HFA, others), levalbuterol (Xopenex HFA), and ipratropium (Atrovent).

Inhaled Steroids: Such as fluticasone (Flovent HFA, Flonase, others) and budesonide (Pulmicort).

Combination Inhalers: These contain an inhaled corticosteroid plus a bronchodilator such as fluticasone and salmeterol (Advair Diskus) or budesonide and formoterol (Symbicort).

Oral Steroids: For severe symptoms or to treat flare-ups.

Phosphodiesterase-4 Inhibitors: Such as roflumilast (Daliresp), specifically for severe COPD associated with chronic bronchitis.

Ayurvedic Approaches

In Ayurveda, COPD is related to "Pranavaha Srotas" and the imbalance of Kapha dosha in the lungs:

Tulsi (Ocimum sanctum): Used for its immunomodulatory and bronchodilator properties.

Licorice (Glycyrrhiza glabra): Used for its soothing and anti-inflammatory effects on the respiratory tract.

Pippali (Piper longum): Known for its rejuvenating and respiratory health-supporting properties.

Vasa (Adhatoda vasica): This herb has expectorant and bronchodilator properties, making it beneficial for respiratory tract disorders.

Yogic Approaches

Yoga offers physical postures, breathing exercises, and meditation that can help improve respiratory health and reduce stress:

Asanas: Postures such as Tadasana (Mountain Pose), Ustrasana (Camel Pose), and Bhujangasana (Cobra Pose) can improve lung capacity and encourage deep breathing.

Pranayama: Breathing exercises like Anulom Vilom (Alternate Nostril Breathing) and Bhastrika (Bellows Breath) can help increase lung capacity and control over breath.

Meditation: Techniques such as mindfulness can help reduce stress and anxiety, which can exacerbate COPD symptoms.

Synergy

Modern medicine, Ayurveda, and Yoga can work together to manage COPD:

Modern medicines provide immediate relief from COPD symptoms, while Ayurvedic herbs may support overall respiratory health.

Yoga postures and pranayama exercises can enhance physical health, improve lung capacity, and promote relaxation.

The stress reduction and mental calming offered by yoga and meditation can complement Modern and Ayurvedic treatments.

Ayurvedic dietary recommendations and lifestyle changes can support overall health and potentially decrease the frequency and severity of COPD symptoms.

It's important for individuals to consult with their healthcare provider or a knowledgeable practitioner before starting or changing any treatment plan. They can provide advice based on individual health conditions and circumstances.

MIGRAINE

Migraine is a type of headache characterized by severe throbbing pain or a pulsing sensation, usually on one side of the head, often accompanied by nausea, vomiting, and extreme sensitivity to light and sound. Here are the Modern medicines, Ayurvedic remedies, and yoga practices that are commonly used for this condition:

Modern Medicine Approaches

In Modern medicine, treatment for migraines aims to relieve symptoms and prevent additional attacks:

Pain Relievers: Aspirin or ibuprofen can help relieve mild migraines. Drugs marketed specifically for migraines, such as the combination of acetaminophen, aspirin and caffeine (Excedrin Migraine), also may ease moderate migraine pain.

Triptans: These are prescription drugs such as sumatriptan (Imitrex, Tosymra) and rizatriptan (Maxalt) that are used to treat severe migraines.

Ergots: Ergotamine and caffeine combination drugs (Migergot, Cafergot) are less effective than triptans.

Anti-nausea Medicines: Certain medications can ease nausea and vomiting associated with migraines. These include chlorpromazine, metoclopramide (Reglan) or prochlorperazine (Compro).

Ayurvedic Approaches

In Ayurveda, migraines are linked to an imbalance of the Tridoshas. Treatment involves balancing these doshas and reducing triggers:

Brahmi (Bacopa monnieri): This herb is often used in Ayurveda to enhance cognitive functioning and reduce stress, both of which can be beneficial for managing migraines.

Shirashuladi Vajra Ras: This is a traditional Ayurvedic medicine used specifically to treat headaches and migraines.

Godanti Bhasma: A mineral-based Ayurvedic treatment that is often used to provide relief from headaches.

Yogic Approaches

Yoga can be beneficial for managing migraines by reducing physical tension and stress, both of which can contribute to migraines:

Asanas: Gentle postures such as Child's Pose (Balasana), Bridge Pose (Setu Bandha Sarvangasana), and Corpse Pose (Savasana) can help reduce muscle tension and promote relaxation.

Pranayama: Breathing exercises such as Anulom Vilom (Alternate Nostril Breathing) and Sheetali (Cooling Breath) can help calm the mind and reduce stress.

Meditation and Relaxation Techniques: Techniques such as mindfulness meditation and progressive muscle relaxation can help manage stress, a common trigger of migraines.

Synergy

The combination of Modern medicine, Ayurveda, and yoga can work together to help manage migraines:

Modern medicine provides immediate symptom relief. Ayurvedic herbs and therapies aim to restore dosha balance, potentially reducing the frequency and severity of migraines.

Yoga postures, breathing exercises, and relaxation techniques can reduce physical tension and manage stress, complementing both Modern and Ayurvedic treatments.

The holistic approach of Ayurveda and yoga—addressing not just physical symptoms but also lifestyle, diet, and mental and emotional health—can enhance overall wellbeing, potentially making one more resilient to migraines.

It's important for individuals to consult with their healthcare provider or a knowledgeable practitioner before starting or changing any treatment plan. They can provide advice based on individual health conditions and circumstances.

INFLAMMATORY BOWEL DISEASE

Inflammatory bowel disease (IBD) includes conditions like Crohn's disease and ulcerative colitis, characterized by chronic inflammation of the digestive tract. Here are the Modern medicines, Ayurvedic remedies, and yoga practices that are commonly used for this condition:

Modern Medicine Approaches

Modern medicine aims to reduce inflammation that can cause symptoms and damage, and to improve long-term prognosis by preventing flare-ups:

Aminosalicylates: Such as sulfasalazine (Azulfidine) and mesalamine (Asacol HD, Delzicol, others). These are often used to treat ulcerative colitis.

Corticosteroids: Such as prednisone and budesonide. These drugs help reduce inflammation.

Immunosuppressants: These drugs reduce inflammation by suppressing the immune response. They include azathioprine (Azasan, Imuran) and mercaptopurine (Purinethol, Purixan).

Biologic Therapies: These drugs target a protein produced by the immune system. They include infliximab (Remicade), adalimumab (Humira) and golimumab (Simponi).

Ayurvedic Approaches

Ayurveda considers IBD as a disease of the large intestine, where Vata dosha is aggravated in the intestines (Purishavaha Srota). Treatment aims to restore balance:

Boswellia (Boswellia serrata): Also known as Indian frankincense, it inhibit 5-lipoxygenase selectively with antiinflammatory and antiarthritic effects and is used in Ayurveda to treat conditions like IBD.

Turmeric (Curcuma longa): The active compound in turmeric, curcumin, curcumin shows anti-inflammatory effect is by attenuating inflammatory response of TNF-α stimulated human endothelial cells by interfering with NF-κB. Furthermore, curcumin is also capable of preventing platelet-derived growth factor (PDGF). This help reduce inflammation in IBD.

Triphala: A traditional Ayurvedic formulation made from three fruits: Amalaki, Bibhitaki, and Haritaki. It's beneficial for overall gut health. Triphala-derived polyphenols such as chebulinic acid are also transformed by the human gut microbiota into metabolites such as urolithins, which have the potential to prevent oxidative damage and inflammation.

Guduchi (Tinospora cordifolia): This herb is used in Ayurveda to support immune health and has anti-inflammatory properties.

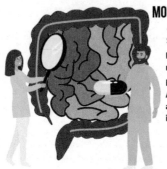

MODERN MEDICINE

Aminosalicylates - Mesalazine, Sulfasalazine

Steroids - Prednisolone, Budesonide

Immunosuppressants - azathioprine, mercaptopurine, suppressess inflammation

Biological therapies - Infliximab, Adalimumab, Golimumab - newer agents and quite effective suppressing bowel inflammation

AYURVEDA

Boswellia Serrata - inhibit 5-lipoxygenase selectively with antiinflammatory

Curcuma Longa - curcumin attenuating inflammatory response of TNF-α stimulated human endothelial cells by interfering with NF-κB.

Trifala - - Amalaki, Bibhitaki, Haritaki - potent anti-inflammatory through polyphenols and urolithins

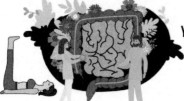

YOGA

Pavanmuktasana - wind-relieving pose
Viparita Karani (legs up the wall pose)
Alternate nostril breathing - anulom vilom
Skull shining breath - Kapal Bhatti
Balasana- child's pose

Yogic Approaches

Yoga can be beneficial for managing IBD by reducing stress and promoting relaxation, which can help ease symptoms and potentially reduce flares:

Asanas: Gentle postures such as Pavanamuktasana (Wind-Relieving Pose), Balasana (Child's Pose), and Viparita Karani (Legs-up-the-Wall Pose) can help soothe the digestive system.

Pranayama: Breathing exercises like Anulom Vilom (Alternate Nostril Breathing) and Kapalabhati (Skull Shining Breath) can help manage stress and stimulate digestion.

Meditation and Relaxation Techniques: Techniques such as mindfulness and progressive muscle relaxation can help manage stress, a common trigger for IBD flares.

Synergy

Modern medicine, Ayurveda, and Yoga can work together to manage IBD:

Modern medicines provide immediate symptom relief and help control inflammation. Ayurvedic herbs and therapies aim to restore dosha balance, potentially reducing the frequency and severity of IBD flares.

Yoga postures and pranayama exercises can help reduce physical tension, manage stress, and promote gut health.

The stress reduction and mental calming offered by yoga and meditation can complement Modern and Ayurvedic treatments.

Ayurvedic dietary recommendations and lifestyle changes can support overall health and potentially decrease the frequency and severity of IBD symptoms.

It's important for individuals to consult with their healthcare provider or a knowledgeable practitioner before starting or changing any treatment plan. They can provide advice based on individual health conditions and circumstances.

IRRITABLE BOWEL SYNDROME

Irritable bowel syndrome (IBS) is a common disorder that affects the large intestine. Symptoms include cramping, abdominal pain, bloating, gas, diarrhoea, and constipation. Here are the Modern medicines, Ayurvedic remedies, and yoga practices that are commonly used for this condition:

Modern Medicine Approaches

Modern medicine treats IBS primarily with medications aimed at relieving the specific symptoms experienced by the individual:

Fiber Supplements: Such as psyllium, fibogel (Metamucil) or methylcellulose (Citrucel) to help control constipation.

Laxatives: For constipation predominant IBS, doctors might suggest magnesium hydroxide oral (Phillips' Milk of Magnesia) or polyethylene glycol (Miralax).

Anti-diarrheal Medications: Over-the-counter medications, such as loperamide (Imodium), can help control diarrhoea.

Antispasmodic Agents: These can help to control colon muscle spasms and reduce abdominal pain. Examples include mebeverine, pippermint oil, dicycloverine hydrochloride, propantheline, hyoscine bromide, Bentyl and Levsin.

Antidepressants: Low doses of tricyclic antidepressants and selective serotonin reuptake inhibitors have been shown to be effective in some people with IBS.

Ayurvedic Approaches

Ayurveda perceives IBS as mainly a disorder of the large intestines and relates it with the vitiation of Vata dosha:

Bilva (Aegle marmelos): The fruit is used to manage diarrhoea, and the root and leaves are used to manage digestive disorders, including IBS.

Hing (Asafoetida): It is commonly used to treat bloating and gas problems. It pacifies Vata and aids in digestion.

Haritaki (Terminalia chebula): It has rejuvenating properties and is used to manage a wide array of health conditions, including IBS.

Musta (Cyperus rotundus): It's used to treat diarrhea and dysentery.

Yogic Approaches

Yoga can help by reducing stress and aiding digestion:

Asanas: Poses like Pavanamuktasana (Wind-Relieving Pose), Ardha Matsyendrasana (Half Lord of the Fishes Pose), and Savasana (Corpse Pose) can help reduce tension and improve digestion.

Pranayama: Breathing exercises like Anulom Vilom (Alternate Nostril Breathing) and Kapalabhati (Skull Shining Breath) can help reduce stress, which is often a trigger for IBS.

Meditation: Techniques such as mindfulness and yoga nidra can help manage stress and anxiety related to IBS.

Synergy

The combination of Modern medicine, Ayurveda, and yoga can provide a holistic approach to managing IBS:

Modern medicines provide symptom relief, Ayurvedic herbs and treatments aim to restore dosha balance, and yoga postures and pranayama exercises can help reduce physical tension and manage stress.

The stress reduction offered by yoga and meditation, as well as the dietary recommendations in Ayurveda, can complement Modern and Ayurvedic treatments.

Ayurvedic lifestyle changes can support overall health, and potentially decrease the frequency and severity of IBS symptoms.

As always, it's important for individuals to consult with their healthcare provider or a knowledgeable practitioner before starting or changing any treatment plan. They can provide advice based on individual health conditions and circumstances.

OBESITY

Obesity is a complex disease involving an excessive amount of body fat. It's a medical problem that increases the risk of other diseases and health problems, such as heart disease, diabetes, high blood pressure and certain cancers. Here are the Modern medicines, Ayurvedic remedies, and yoga practices that are commonly used for this condition:

Modern Medicine Approaches

Modern medicine aims to reduce body weight and treat the accompanying health risks:

Behavioral treatment (Diet, physical activity & behaviour changes): This is a useful approach for weight loss and can enhance weight loss when combined with drug therapy.

Weight Loss Medications: Such as Orlistat (Alli, Xenical), Lorcaserin (Belviq), Phentermine and topiramate (Qsymia), Bupropion and naltrexone (Contrave), and Liraglutide (Saxenda).

Weight-loss Surgery (bariatric surgery): Surgery is usually recommended for individuals with a BMI of 40 or more, or those with a BMI of 35 or more who have weight-related problems.

Ayurvedic Approaches

Ayurveda suggests a combination of diet, exercise, and specific herbal supplements for managing obesity:

Guggul (Commiphora mukul): It is used to lower bad cholesterol and increase good cholesterol. It also enhances the function of the thyroid gland and aids in weight loss.

Garcinia Cambogia: Hydroxycitric acid, the active ingredient in the fruit's rind, has boosted fat-burning and cut back appetite in studies.

Triphala: A mix of Ayurvedic fruits, including Amalaki, Bibhitaki, and Haritaki, Triphala is an effective laxative that also supports digestion and detoxification.

Cumin: Cumin is believed to enhance the metabolic rate and thus aid weight loss.

Yogic Approaches

Yoga can be an effective tool to manage weight, stress, and improve overall physical fitness:

Asanas: Poses like Surya Namaskar (Sun Salutation), Virabhadrasana (Warrior Pose), and Trikonasana (Triangle Pose) can help burn fat, strengthen muscles, and improve flexibility. Mandukasana is good for belly fat , particularly when combinesd with Kapalb Bhatti.

Pranayama: Breathing exercises like Kapala Bhati (Skull Shining Breath) can help increase metabolic rate and aid in weight loss.You can start with 1 deep breath in with 1 per second breath out (60 per minute and go up to 90 per minute). Need to do regularly every day for at least 5 minutes to see the effect.

Meditation: Techniques such as mindfulness and yoga nidra can help manage stress and anxiety, which can lead to overeating and weight gain.

Synergy

The combination of Modern medicine, Ayurveda, and yoga can provide a holistic approach to managing obesity:

Modern or Modern medicines and surgical approaches provide symptom relief and immediate weight loss, Ayurvedic herbs and treatments aim to boost metabolism and aid digestion, and yoga postures and pranayama exercises can help reduce physical tension and manage stress.

The stress reduction offered by yoga and meditation, as well as the dietary recommendations in Ayurveda, can complement Modern and Ayurvedic treatments.

Ayurvedic lifestyle changes can support overall health, and potentially decrease weight and maintain a healthy weight.

As always, it's important for individuals to consult with their healthcare provider or a knowledgeable practitioner before starting or changing any treatment plan. They can provide advice based on individual health conditions and circumstances.

CHRONIC ECZEMA

Eczema, also known as atopic dermatitis, is a condition that causes inflamed, itchy, cracked, and rough skin. Here are the Modern medicines, Ayurvedic remedies, and yoga practices that are commonly used for this condition:

Modern Medicine Approaches

Modern medicine aims to control the itching, reduce inflammation, prevent outbreaks, and heal the skin:

Topical corticosteroids: These medications, such as hydrocortisone, are used to control inflammation and reduce immune system activity in milder eczema. Clobetasone for moderate and Betamethasone for severe eczema.

Topical calcineurin inhibitors: These include medications like pimecrolimus (Elidel) and tacrolimus (Protopic).

Systemic corticosteroids: In severe cases, oral corticosteroids such as prednisone may be used.

Biologic drugs: Infliximab, Dupilumab (Dupixent) is an injectable medication that works by controlling the immune response.

Ayurvedic Approaches

In Ayurveda, eczema is often viewed as a condition that is primarily due to imbalance in the Vata and Pitta doshas:

Neem (Azadirachta indica): This herb is renowned for its anti-inflammatory, antibacterial, and antifungal properties.

Turmeric (Curcuma longa): The active ingredient, curcumin, has anti-inflammatory and antioxidant properties.

Aloe Vera: It can provide relief from itching and inflammation and improve skin healing.

Ghee: Ghee, especially when processed with certain herbs, is used topically to soothe the skin and promote healing.

Yogic Approaches

Yoga can help manage the stress and anxiety often associated with chronic skin conditions like eczema:

Asanas: Gentle postures like Shishuasana (Child's Pose), Viparita Karani (Legs Up the Wall Pose), and Shavasana (Corpse Pose) can help soothe the nervous system.

Pranayama: Breathing practices like Anulom Vilom (Alternate Nostril Breathing) and Bhramari (Bee Breath) can help reduce stress.

Meditation: Mindfulness meditation can help reduce stress, potentially lessening flare-ups.

Synergy

Modern medicine, Ayurveda, and Yoga can work together to manage eczema:

Modern medicines provide immediate symptom relief and manage acute flare-ups. Ayurvedic herbs aim to correct the underlying dosha imbalance and promote skin health.

Yoga postures and pranayama exercises can help manage stress, which can be a trigger for eczema flare-ups.

The stress reduction and mental calming offered by yoga and meditation can complement Modern and Ayurvedic treatments.

Ayurvedic dietary recommendations and lifestyle changes can support overall skin health and potentially decrease the frequency and severity of eczema symptoms.

As always, it's important for individuals to consult with their healthcare provider or a knowledgeable practitioner before starting or changing any treatment plan. They can provide advice based on individual health conditions and circumstances.

DYSMENORRHOEA

Dysmenorrhea is the medical term for pain with menstruation, commonly known as menstrual cramps. Here are the Modern medicines, Ayurvedic remedies, and yoga practices that are commonly used for this condition:

Modern Medicine Approaches

Modern medicine aims to relieve the pain and address the underlying cause, if it is known:

Nonsteroidal anti-inflammatory drugs (NSAIDs): Over-the-counter NSAIDs, such as ibuprofen (Advil, Motrin IB, others) and naproxen sodium (Aleve), at regular doses can relieve the pain of dysmenorrhea.

Hormonal birth control: Oral contraceptives, patches, vaginal rings, injections, and intrauterine devices can lessen menstrual pain.

Antidepressants: Certain antidepressants, such as a class of drugs called selective serotonin reuptake inhibitors (SSRIs), may be helpful in some cases.

Ayurvedic Approaches

Ayurveda suggests a combination of herbs, diet, and lifestyle modifications for managing dysmenorrhea:

Shatavari (Asparagus racemosus): Known as the 'Queen of Herbs' for female health, Shatavari can balance the hormonal system and reduce menstrual pain.

Ashoka (Saraca Asoca): The bark of the Ashoka tree is used to relieve menstrual pain due to its uterine tonic properties.

Ginger (Zingiber officinale): Ginger is well known for its anti-inflammatory and analgesic properties, and can be helpful in relieving menstrual pain.

Fennel (Foeniculum vulgare): Fennel is believed to reduce the intensity of dysmenorrhea, and has antispasmodic and analgesic properties.

Yogic Approaches

Yoga can help by reducing stress and tension and improving the function of the reproductive system:

Asanas: Poses like Janu Sirsasana (Head-to-Knee Forward Bend), Pasasana (Noose Pose), and Savasana (Corpse Pose) can help reduce tension and improve the functioning of the reproductive system.

Pranayama: Breathing exercises like Anulom Vilom (Alternate Nostril Breathing) and Kapalabhati (Skull Shining Breath) can help reduce stress and promote relaxation.

Meditation: Techniques such as mindfulness and yoga nidra can help manage stress and anxiety related to dysmenorrhea.

Synergy

The combination of Modern medicine, Ayurveda, and yoga can provide a holistic approach to managing dysmenorrhea:

Modern medicines provide immediate symptom relief, Ayurvedic herbs and treatments aim to restore balance and manage pain, and yoga postures and pranayama exercises can help reduce physical tension and manage stress.

The stress reduction offered by yoga and meditation, as well as the dietary recommendations in Ayurveda, can complement Modern and Ayurvedic treatments.

Ayurvedic lifestyle changes can support overall health, and potentially decrease the severity of dysmenorrhea symptoms.

As always, it's important for individuals to consult with their healthcare provider or a knowledgeable practitioner before starting or changing any treatment plan. They can provide advice based on individual health conditions and circumstances.

CHRONIC FATIGUE SYNDROME

Chronic Fatigue Syndrome (CFS), also known as Myalgic Encephalomyelitis (ME), is a complex disorder characterized by extreme fatigue that can't be explained by any underlying medical condition. Here are the Modern medicines, Ayurvedic remedies, and yoga practices that are commonly used for this condition:

Modern Medicine Approaches

There's currently no specific treatment for CFS, but certain medications and therapies can help manage symptoms:

Antidepressants: Certain types of antidepressants can help improve sleep and relieve the pain and fatigue associated with CFS.

Sleeping pills: In some cases, doctors may recommend medications to help improve sleep.

Physiotherapy (physical therapy): A physical therapist can help develop a personalised exercise program that could help improve strength and functioning.

Ayurvedic Approaches

In Ayurveda, CFS is often viewed as a condition that is primarily due to an imbalance in the Vata dosha:

Ashwagandha (Withania somnifera): This adaptogenic herb is often used to help the body resist physical and mental stress.

Brahmi (Bacopa monnieri): Brahmi is known for its brain-boosting and stress-relieving properties.

Amalaki (Emblica officinalis): Also known as Indian gooseberry, Amalaki is a rejuvenative herb that helps boost immunity and reduce fatigue.

Shatavari (Asparagus racemosus): This herb is used to rejuvenate the body, strengthen the immune system, and improve physical strength.

Yogic Approaches

Yoga can help manage the stress and anxiety often associated with CFS:

Asanas: Gentle postures like Tadasana (Mountain Pose), Balasana (Child's Pose), and Savasana (Corpse Pose) can help to reduce physical tension and promote relaxation.

Pranayama: Breathing practices like Nadi Shodhana (Alternate Nostril Breathing) and Ujjayi (Victorious Breath or Ocean Breath) can help to balance the nervous system and reduce stress.

Meditation: Mindfulness meditation can help manage stress and anxiety, potentially improving the symptoms of CFS.

Synergy

Modern medicine, Ayurveda, and yoga can work together to manage CFS:

Modern medicines can provide immediate symptom relief, while Ayurvedic herbs aim to correct the underlying dosha imbalance and strengthen the body.

Yoga postures and pranayama exercises can help manage stress and enhance physical strength and energy.

The relaxation and stress reduction offered by yoga and meditation can complement Modern and Ayurvedic treatments.

Ayurvedic dietary recommendations and lifestyle changes can support overall health and potentially decrease the severity of CFS symptoms.

As always, it's important for individuals to consult with their healthcare provider or a knowledgeable practitioner before starting or changing any treatment plan. They can provide advice based on individual health conditions and circumstances.

SYSTEMIC LUPUS ERYTHEMATOSUS (SLE)

Systemic Lupus Erythematosus (SLE), or lupus, is an autoimmune disease in which the immune system attacks its own tissues, causing widespread inflammation and tissue damage. Here are the Modern medicines, Ayurvedic remedies, and yoga practices that are commonly used for this condition:

Modern Medicine Approaches

The goal of treatment in lupus is to minimize symptoms, reduce inflammation and pain, and prevent damage to organs:

Nonsteroidal anti-inflammatory drugs (NSAIDs): These medications, such as ibuprofen and naproxen, can control inflammation and are often used to treat mild symptoms of lupus.

Antimalarial drugs: Medications such as hydroxychloroquine (Plaquenil) are sometimes used to manage symptoms of lupus.

Corticosteroids: These are powerful anti-inflammatory drugs, such as prednisone, used to control severe symptoms and organ-threatening disease.

Immunosuppressants: Drugs like methotrexate, azathioprine, mycophenolate, and cyclophosphamide are used in severe cases to suppress the immune system.

Ayurvedic Approaches

In Ayurveda, SLE is considered as an imbalance in all the three doshas - Vata, Pitta, and Kapha. It aims at immune modulation and the management of symptoms:

Giloy (Tinospora cordifolia): It's a potent immunomodulator and can help control the abnormal immune response in lupus.

Ashwagandha (Withania somnifera): This adaptogenic herb is known to reduce stress and inflammation.

Turmeric (Curcuma longa): The active ingredient, curcumin, has anti-inflammatory properties and can help manage inflammation in lupus.

Amla (Emblica officinalis): Also known as Indian Gooseberry, Amla is a potent antioxidant and helps in enhancing the body's immunity.

Yogic Approaches

Yoga can help manage stress, enhance mood, and improve the quality of life in patients with lupus:

Asanas: Gentle postures like Balasana (Child's Pose), Viparita Karani (Legs-Up-the-Wall Pose), and Shavasana (Corpse Pose) can help to reduce stress and promote relaxation.

Pranayama: Breathing exercises such as Anulom Vilom (Alternate Nostril Breathing) and Bhramari (Bee Breath) can help to balance the nervous system and reduce stress.

Meditation: Mindfulness meditation can help manage stress and anxiety, potentially improving overall wellbeing.

Synergy

Combining Modern medicine, Ayurveda, and yoga can provide a holistic approach to managing lupus:

Modern medicines provide immediate symptom relief and control severe symptoms, while Ayurvedic herbs aim to correct the underlying dosha imbalance and strengthen the immune system.

Yoga postures and pranayama exercises can help manage stress and enhance physical strength and energy, which are often affected in lupus.

The relaxation and stress reduction offered by yoga and meditation can complement Modern and Ayurvedic treatments.

Ayurvedic dietary recommendations and lifestyle changes can support overall health and potentially decrease the severity of lupus symptoms.

As always, it's important for individuals to consult with their healthcare provider or a knowledgeable practitioner before starting or changing any treatment plan. They can provide advice based on individual health conditions and circumstances.

MULTIPLE SCLEROSIS

Multiple sclerosis (MS) is a potentially disabling disease of the brain and spinal cord where the immune system attacks the protective sheath (myelin) that covers nerve fibres. Here are the Modern medicines, Ayurvedic remedies, and yoga practices that are commonly used for this condition:

Modern Medicine Approaches

The goal of treatment in MS is to manage symptoms, reduce inflammation, slow the progression of the disease, and improve quality of life:

Corticosteroids: These are powerful anti-inflammatory drugs used to reduce inflammation during severe attacks.

Beta interferons: These drugs, including Avonex and Betaseron, are often the first line of treatment and can reduce the frequency and severity of relapses.

Glatiramer acetate (Copaxone): This medication helps block your immune system's attack on myelin.

Physiotherapy (Physical therapy): This can help manage symptoms like pain, stiffness, and trouble moving.

Ayurvedic Approaches

In Ayurveda, MS is often viewed as a Vata disorder, but it can also involve imbalances in the other doshas:

Ashwagandha (Withania somnifera): This herb is an adaptogen, has some neuroregenerative effect, adaptogenic properties helps the body manage stress, and it also has anti-inflammatory properties.

Brahmi (Bacopa monnieri): Brahmi is known for its neuroprotective properties and can help improve cognitive function.

Turmeric (Curcuma longa): The active ingredient, curcumin, has anti-inflammatory and antioxidant properties that may help reduce inflammation and oxidative stress.

Amalaki (Emblica officinalis): Also known as Indian gooseberry, Amalaki is a potent antioxidant that can help strengthen the immune system.

Yogic Approaches

Yoga can help manage stress, increase mobility, and improve quality of life in patients with MS:

Asanas: Gentle postures like Tadasana (Mountain Pose), Vrikshasana (Tree Pose), and Setu Bandha Sarvangasana (Bridge Pose) can help improve balance, strength, and flexibility.

Pranayama: Breathing exercises such as Anulom Vilom (Alternate Nostril Breathing) and Bhramari (Bee Breath) can help to balance the nervous system and reduce stress.

Meditation: Techniques such as mindfulness and guided imagery can help manage stress, reduce symptoms of anxiety and depression, and improve overall wellbeing.

Synergy

The combination of Modern medicine, Ayurveda, and yoga can provide a comprehensive approach to managing MS:

Modern medicines can provide immediate symptom relief and slow disease progression, while Ayurvedic herbs aim to correct the underlying dosha imbalance and strengthen the body.

Yoga postures and pranayama exercises can help manage stress, improve physical function, and enhance quality of life, which are often affected in MS.

The relaxation and stress reduction offered by yoga and meditation can complement Modern and Ayurvedic treatments.

Ayurvedic dietary recommendations and lifestyle changes can support overall health and potentially decrease the severity of MS symptoms.

As always, it's important for individuals to consult with their healthcare provider or a knowledgeable practitioner before starting or changing any treatment plan. They can provide advice based on individual health conditions and circumstances.

FIBROMYALGIA

Fibromyalgia is a neuropathic pain disorder characterised by widespread musculoskeletal pain accompanied by fatigue, sleep, memory and mood issues. The pain quite severe as it is neuropathic and researchers have found that fibromyalgia amplifies painful sensations by affecting the way your brain and spinal cord process painful and non-painful signals. It is believed to be due to neurotransmitter imbalance in brain and spinal cord. Here are the Modern medicines, Ayurvedic remedies, and yoga practices that are commonly used for this condition:

Modern Medicine Approaches

The goal of treatment in fibromyalgia is to manage symptoms and improve quality of life:

Pain relievers: Over-the-counter pain relievers such as paracecamol (acetaminophen), ibuprofen, or naproxen sodium may be helpful on some occasions.

Antidepressants: Drugs like Duloxetine (Cymbalta) or Milnacipran (Savella) may help ease the pain and fatigue associated with fibromyalgia.

Antiseizure drugs: Medications designed to treat epilepsy, like Gabapentin (Neurontin) or Pregabalin (Lyrica), are often useful in reducing certain types of pain.

Ayurvedic Approaches

In Ayurveda, fibromyalgia is often seen as a Vata imbalance. Here are some herbal remedies that might help:

Ginkgo Biloba - helps to rebalance the neurotransmitters and found helpful in scientific study to reduce symptoms of fibromyalgia ,, particularly when used with Coenzyme Q 10.

Guarna – is a neurostimulant and tends to help fatigue which is other predominant symptom in fibromyalgia.

Super Nerve Power – It's a combination of Ginkgo Biloba, Guarna, Green Tea extract , Beet Root Extract, Phosphodiesterase inhibitor and Coenzyme Q10. The combination is reported to help a lot of patients of fibromyalgia due to help with severe neuropathic pain, fatigue, and brain fog by primarily addressing the root cause.

Ashwagandha (Withania somnifera): Ashwagandha is adaptogenic tonic that nourishes the nerves, also builds core energy , and is known for its stress-lowering effects, which can aid in the sleep issues and anxiety often associated with fibromyalgia.

Boswellia (Boswellia serrata): Known for its anti-inflammatory properties, it can help reduce pain and swelling.

Turmeric (Curcuma longa): Its active ingredient, curcumin, has anti-inflammatory properties and can aid in managing inflammation.

Shatavari (Asparagus racemosus): This is often used to soothe Vata imbalances, and it's also known to have anti-inflammatory properties.

Yogic Approaches

Yoga can help manage pain, improve mood, and enhance overall wellbeing:

Asanas: Gentle stretching poses like Tadasana (Mountain Pose), Balasana (Child's Pose), or Viparita Karani (Legs-up-the-Wall Pose) can be beneficial.

Pranayama: Breathing exercises like Anulom Vilom (Alternate Nostril Breathing) and Kapalbhati (Skull Shining Breath) can help manage stress and promote relaxation.

Meditation: Techniques such as mindfulness meditation can help manage stress and anxiety, often improving overall wellbeing.

Synergy

The combination of Modern medicine, Ayurveda, and yoga can provide a comprehensive approach to managing fibromyalgia:

Modern medicines can provide immediate symptom relief, while Ayurvedic herbs aim to correct the underlying dosha imbalance and strengthen the body.

Yoga postures and pranayama exercises can help manage stress, improve physical function, and enhance quality of life.

The relaxation and stress reduction offered by yoga and meditation can complement Modern and Ayurvedic treatments.

Ayurvedic dietary recommendations and lifestyle changes can support overall health and potentially decrease the severity of fibromyalgia symptoms.

As always, it's important for individuals to consult with their healthcare provider or a knowledgeable practitioner before starting or changing any treatment plan. They can provide advice based on individual health conditions and circumstances.

HYPOTHYROIDISM

Hypothyroidism is a condition in which the thyroid gland doesn't produce enough thyroid hormones. It's often due to an underlying issue such as Hashimoto's disease. Here are the Modern medicines, Ayurvedic remedies, and yoga practices that are commonly used for this condition:

Modern Medicine Approaches

The main treatment for hypothyroidism is hormone replacement therapy:

Levothyroxine: This is the most commonly prescribed medication for hypothyroidism. It's a synthetic form of thyroxine (T4), one of the hormones the thyroid gland produces.

Ayurvedic Approaches

In Ayurveda, hypothyroidism is often associated with an imbalance in Kapha dosha. Here are some herbal remedies that might help:

Guggul (Commiphora mukul): It's traditionally used for conditions linked to obesity and high cholesterol, and it might help stimulate thyroid function.

Ashwagandha (Withania somnifera): Ashwagandha can support thyroid function by helping the body adapt to stress and supporting immune function. Said to have some effect on Hypothalamo pituitary axis.

Kanchanar (Bauhinia variegate): Kanchanar is traditionally used for thyroid health, particularly for conditions associated with hypothyroidism and goiter.

Triphala: A combination of three fruits, Amalaki (Emblica officinalis), Bibhitaki (Terminalia bellirica), and Haritaki (Terminalia chebula), Triphala is known for its detoxifying and rejuvenating properties.

Yogic Approaches

Yoga can help manage symptoms, reduce stress, and enhance overall wellbeing:

Asanas: Poses that stimulate the throat area can be beneficial, such as Sarvangasana (Shoulder Stand), Halasana (Plow Pose), and Matsyasana (Fish Pose).

Pranayama: Breathing exercises like Ujjayi (Victorious Breath) and Kapalbhati (Skull Shining Breath) can help stimulate the thyroid gland.

Meditation: Techniques such as mindfulness meditation can help manage stress and support overall wellbeing.

Synergy

The combination of Modern medicine, Ayurveda, and yoga can provide a comprehensive approach to managing hypothyroidism:

Levothyroxine provides the body with the thyroid hormone it's lacking, which is crucial for metabolism and energy levels.

Ayurvedic herbs aim to balance the doshas and stimulate the thyroid gland to improve its function.

Yoga poses stimulate the thyroid gland, while pranayama and meditation help manage stress and support overall health.

Ayurvedic dietary recommendations can further support thyroid health. For example, seaweed and other iodine-rich foods can support thyroid function, as the thyroid uses iodine to make its hormones.

As always, it's important for individuals to consult with their healthcare provider or a knowledgeable practitioner before starting or changing any treatment plan. They can provide advice based on individual health conditions and circumstances.

HYPERTHYROIDISM

Hyperthyroidism is a condition where the thyroid gland is overactive and produces too much of its hormone. The most common cause is Graves' disease, an autoimmune disorder. Here are the Modern medicines, Ayurvedic remedies, and yoga practices that are commonly used for this condition:

Modern Medicine Approaches

Hyperthyroidism is usually treated with medications, radioactive iodine, or surgery:

Beta Blockers: Such as propranolol, to manage rapid heart rate and anxiety.

Anti-thyroid Medications: Propylthiouracil and methimazole to reduce symptoms by preventing the thyroid from producing excess amounts of hormone.

Radioactive Iodine: It's used to shrink the thyroid gland and limit its hormone production.

Ayurvedic Approaches

In Ayurveda, hyperthyroidism is seen as an imbalance in Pitta dosha. Here are some herbal remedies that might help:

Bugleweed (Lycopusvirginica): It's known for its ability to help manage mild hyperthyroidism.

Lemon Balm (Melissa officinalis): It can help inhibit the binding of antibodies to the thyroid in Graves' disease.

Shatavari (Asparagus racemosus): This is often used to balance Pitta and reduce inflammation.

Brahmi (Bacopa monnieri): It has been used to improve thyroid hormone levels and reduce anxiety.

Yogic Approaches

Yoga can help manage symptoms, reduce stress, and enhance overall wellbeing:

Asanas: Gentle postures like Shavasana (Corpse Pose), Marjaryasana (Cat Pose), and Balasana (Child's Pose) can be beneficial.

Pranayama: Breathing exercises like Anulom Vilom (Alternate Nostril Breathing) and Bhramari (Bee Breath) can help manage stress and support overall health.

Meditation: Techniques such as mindfulness meditation can help manage stress and support overall wellbeing.

Synergy

The combination of Modern medicine, Ayurveda, and yoga can provide a comprehensive approach to managing hyperthyroidism:

Modern medications can rapidly control the symptoms, while radioactive iodine therapy or surgery can provide a long-term solution.

Ayurvedic herbs can help balance the underlying dosha imbalance and provide a holistic approach to treatment.

Yoga can aid in stress management, improve physical function, and enhance the quality of life.

Ayurvedic dietary recommendations and lifestyle changes can support overall health and potentially decrease the severity of hyperthyroidism symptoms.

As always, it's important for individuals to consult with their healthcare provider or a knowledgeable practitioner before starting or changing any treatment plan. They can provide advice based on individual health conditions and circumstances.

ANXIETY DISORDER

Anxiety disorders are characterized by a variety of symptoms, including excessive fear, restlessness, and often physical symptoms like a fast heart rate. Here's how Modern medicine, Ayurveda, and yoga can be used together for a holistic approach to managing anxiety disorders:

Modern Medicine Approaches

Medications, psychotherapy, and lifestyle changes are often part of an integrated treatment plan for anxiety:

Selective Serotonin Reuptake Inhibitors (SSRIs): Such as fluoxetine and sertraline. These help to increase the level of serotonin, a neurotransmitter associated with mood regulation, in the brain.

Benzodiazepines: Such as diazepam and alprazolam. These are used for their fast-acting relief of acute symptoms, as they help to calm the nervous system.

Psychotherapy: Cognitive-behavioural therapy (CBT) is especially useful for treating anxiety disorders. It helps patients identify and manage the thoughts that cause anxiety.

Ayurvedic Approaches

Ayurveda views anxiety as a result of an imbalance in the Vata dosha. Here are some remedies that might help:

Ashwagandha (Withania somnifera): This adaptogenic herb is used to relieve stress and promote relaxation.

Brahmi (Bacopa monnieri): Brahmi is used to reduce anxiety and improve cognitive function.

Jatamansi (Nardostachys jatamansi): This herb is used for its calming and sleep-enhancing properties.

Pippali (Piper longum): Pippali is used to balance Vata and Kapha doshas and strengthen the nervous system.

Yogic Approaches

Yoga, pranayama, and meditation are known for their stress-relieving and calming effects:

Asanas: Poses like Child's Pose (Balasana), Bridge Pose (Setu Bandha Sarvangasana), and Legs-Up-The-Wall Pose (Viparita Karani) can help to relax the body and mind.

Pranayama: Breathing techniques like Alternate Nostril Breathing (Anulom Vilom) and Bee Breath (Bhramari Pranayama) can help to calm the mind.

Meditation: Mindfulness and Transcendental Meditation are effective techniques for reducing anxiety.

Synergy

The combination of these three modalities can provide a comprehensive and holistic approach to managing anxiety:

Modern medications can help to manage acute symptoms of anxiety, and psychotherapy can provide tools to deal with triggering situations.

Ayurvedic herbs can help to balance the underlying dosha imbalance and provide overall calming and rejuvenating effects.

Yoga and meditation can help to manage daily stress levels, enhance self-awareness, and promote a sense of peace and well-being.

It's essential for anyone suffering from an anxiety disorder to seek professional advice before starting or changing any treatment plan. A healthcare provider can offer guidance based on individual health conditions and circumstances.

DEPRESSION

Depression is a mental health disorder characterized by a persistently depressed mood or loss of interest in activities, causing significant impairment in daily life. A combination of Modern medicine, Ayurveda, and Yoga can provide a comprehensive approach to manage depression.

Modern Medicine Approaches

Selective Serotonin Reuptake Inhibitors (SSRIs): These include medications like fluoxetine and sertraline. SSRIs are a common type of antidepressant that can help increase the level of serotonin in the brain.

Serotonin and Norepinephrine Reuptake Inhibitors (SNRIs): These include venlafaxine and duloxetine. SNRIs can increase levels of serotonin and norepinephrine in the brain to boost mood.

Psychotherapy: Cognitive-behavioural therapy (CBT) and other types of therapy can help a person identify and change thought patterns that lead to feelings of depression.

Ayurvedic Approaches

In Ayurveda, depression is often attributed to an imbalance in the three doshas, but particularly to increased Vata.

Ashwagandha (Withania somnifera): It is an adaptogenic herb that can help the body cope with daily stress, and optimize energy levels.

Brahmi (Bacopa monnieri): It has been traditionally used to enhance cognitive abilities, reduce stress, and promote relaxation.

Jatamansi (Nardostachys jatamansi): This herb is known for its calming effects and ability to promote quality sleep.

Saffron (Crocus sativus): It can improve mood and may be as effective as certain antidepressants in treating depression.

Yogic Approaches

Yoga and meditation have been found to reduce symptoms of depression by decreasing stress levels and promoting a sense of wellbeing:

Asanas: Poses such as Child's Pose (Balasana), Bridge Pose (Setu Bandha Sarvangasana), and Downward-Facing Dog (Adho Mukha Svanasana) can release tension and improve mood.

Pranayama: Breathing exercises like Alternate Nostril Breathing (Anulom Vilom) and Skull Shining Breath (Kapalbhati) can help to balance energy and promote a calm mind.

Meditation: Techniques such as mindfulness and loving-kindness meditation can help shift thought patterns and alleviate symptoms of depression.

Synergy

By using all three approaches, one can gain control over depression from various angles:

Modern medication can help quickly reduce severe symptoms and restore biochemistry balance in the brain.

Ayurvedic herbs can address the imbalances of the doshas and promote physical and mental health.

Yoga and meditation can provide natural mood enhancement, help manage stress, and cultivate a positive mindset.

As always, individuals should consult with their healthcare provider or a knowledgeable practitioner before starting any new treatment or making any changes to their existing treatment plan. They can provide advice based on individual health conditions and circumstances.

ATTENTION DEFICIT HYPERACTIVITY (ADHD)

Attention Deficit Hyperactivity Disorder (ADHD) is a neurodevelopmental disorder characterized by inattention, hyperactivity, and impulsivity that interferes with functioning or development. A combination of Modern medicine, Ayurveda, and Yoga can offer a holistic approach to managing ADHD:

Modern Medicine Approaches

Stimulant Medications: These include medications like methylphenidate and amphetamines, which increase the levels of certain chemicals in the brain that help with thinking and attention.

Non-stimulant Medications: These include medications like atomoxetine, guanfacine, and clonidine which work differently than stimulants to control ADHD symptoms.

Behavioural Therapy: This involves working with a therapist to learn new behaviours to replace behaviours that don't work or cause problems.

Ayurvedic Approaches

In Ayurveda, ADHD is typically associated with imbalances in Vata. So, treatments focus on reducing Vata and increasing Kapha:

Brahmi (Bacopa monnieri): It is used to enhance memory and cognition and to alleviate stress and anxiety.

Mandukaparni (Centella asiatica): It is also known as Gotu Kola, used for its positive effects on mental health.

Shankhpushpi (Convolvulus pluricaulis): This plant is used for its potential memory-boosting and neuroprotective effects.

Vacha (Acorus calamus): This herb is used for its beneficial effects on cognitive function and attention.

Yogic Approaches

Yoga and meditation have been found to help children with ADHD by improving their ability to remain calm, focus, and follow instructions:

Asanas: Poses like Tree Pose (Vrikshasana), Warrior II (Virabhadrasana II), and Crow Pose (Kakasana) can help improve balance, concentration, and calmness.

Pranayama: Breathing exercises like Belly Breathing (Diaphragmatic Breathing) and Cooling Breath (Sitali Pranayama) can help to control energy levels and promote calmness.

Meditation: Techniques like mindfulness can help improve focus and reduce impulsivity and hyperactivity.

Synergy

The combination of these three modalities provides a comprehensive approach to managing ADHD:

Modern medications can help manage the symptoms of ADHD effectively and can be crucial for some individuals in managing daily tasks and activities.

Ayurvedic herbs can help balance the doshas and provide a holistic approach to managing ADHD symptoms.

Yoga and meditation can help children with ADHD enhance their ability to concentrate, reduce impulsivity, and improve their capacity for self-control.

As always, the management of ADHD should be individualized, and decisions regarding treatment must be made in consultation with a healthcare provider. They can provide advice based on individual health conditions and circumstances.

INSOMNIA

Insomnia is a common sleep disorder that can make it hard to fall asleep, hard to stay asleep, or cause early morning awakening. Combining Modern medicine, Ayurveda, and Yoga can provide a holistic approach to manage insomnia:

Modern Medicine Approaches

Benzodiazepines: These include medications like temazepam and lorazepam. They act on the central nervous system to produce sedation and muscle relaxation.

Non-Benzodiazepines (Z-Drugs): These include zolpidem, zopiclone, and eszopiclone. They are sedative-hypnotic drugs that have similar effects to benzodiazepines but a different chemical structure.

Antidepressants: Some antidepressants, such as trazodone, are often used off-label to treat insomnia.

Cognitive Behavioral Therapy for Insomnia (CBT-I): This type of therapy helps you change thoughts and behaviors that cause or worsen sleep problems with habits that promote sound sleep.

Ayurvedic Approaches

In Ayurveda, insomnia is often associated with an imbalance in the Vata dosha. Various herbs are used to calm the mind and promote sleep:

Ashwagandha (Withania somnifera): It's an adaptogen known to reduce stress and promote sleep.

Brahmi (Bacopa monnieri): It's used to relieve stress and anxiety, improve cognition and promote relaxation.

Jatamansi (Nardostachys jatamansi): Known for its calming effects and ability to promote quality sleep.

Valerian (Valeriana officinalis): It helps to relax the central nervous system and promotes a sense of tranquility.

Yogic Approaches

Yoga and meditation can help reduce stress and anxiety, promoting better sleep:

Asanas: Poses like Child's Pose (Balasana), Legs-Up-The-Wall Pose (Viparita Karani), and Corpse Pose (Savasana) can promote relaxation and aid sleep.

Pranayama: Breathing exercises like the Cooling Breath (Shitali Pranayama) and Bee Breath (Bhramari Pranayama) can help soothe the nervous system and facilitate sleep.

Meditation and Yoga Nidra: Mindfulness meditation and Yoga Nidra can help the mind relax and prepare the body for sleep.

Synergy

The combination of these three approaches provides a comprehensive method to managing insomnia:

Modern medications can be useful for short-term relief from severe insomnia.

Ayurvedic herbs can help soothe the nervous system and promote better sleep quality in the long run.

Yoga and meditation can help manage stress and anxiety, both of which are common causes of insomnia.

The synergy of these treatments can be tailored to the individual's needs and provide a holistic approach to better sleep. As always, consult with a healthcare provider or knowledgeable practitioner to understand what treatment combination might work best.

ANOREXIA NERVOSA

Anorexia nervosa is a psychological eating disorder characterized by an intense fear of gaining weight and a distorted body image that results in self-imposed starvation and excessive weight loss. It often coexists with other disorders like anxiety, depression, and insomnia. Managing anorexia nervosa can require a multi-modal approach combining Modern medicine, Ayurveda, and Yoga.

Modern Medicine Approaches

Nutritional Therapy: A professional specialist dietitian provides guidance to ensure the individual is receiving the necessary nutrients. Tube feeding is done when nutritional compromise happens, and this provides macronutrients like protein, carbohydrate and fat as well as micronutrients.

Psychotropic Medications: Certain selective serotonin reuptake inhibitors (SSRIs) like fluoxetine and antipsychotic medications such as olanzapine may be used to help manage the underlying anxiety and obsessive thoughts related to food and body image.

Cognitive Behavioural Therapy (CBT): This therapy can help the individual develop a healthier relationship with food and their body image.

Ayurvedic Approaches

In Ayurveda, anorexia nervosa is often associated with disturbances in the bodily humors (doshas), particularly Vata.

Ashwagandha (Withania somnifera): It's an adaptogen known to reduce stress and anxiety, which can indirectly support healthier eating behaviors.

Shatavari (Asparagus racemosus): This herb is known to balance pitta and vata doshas and may promote digestive health.

Chyawanprash: A traditional Ayurvedic herbal jam, including Amla (Indian gooseberry) and many other herbs, which is known to promote overall strength and immunity.

Yogic Approaches

Yoga and meditation can help reduce stress and improve body image, which can be beneficial in managing anorexia nervosa:

Asanas: Gentle yoga poses like Mountain Pose (Tadasana), Tree Pose (Vrikshasana), and Warrior II (Virabhadrasana II) can help to promote a sense of groundedness and body awareness.

Pranayama: Breathing exercises like Equal Breathing (Sama Vritti) and Lion's Breath (Simhasana) can help reduce anxiety.

Meditation and Mindfulness practices: These can help improve the mind-body connection and promote a healthier body image.

Synergy

Modern medication and therapy can address the immediate psychiatric needs, nutritional deficiencies, and cognitive distortions associated with anorexia nervosa.

Ayurvedic herbs may support overall strength, promote a healthy digestive system, and help balance the disturbed doshas.

Yoga and meditation can help improve mental well-being, reduce anxiety, and foster a healthier body image.

Remember that anorexia nervosa is a serious condition that should be managed by a healthcare provider or a team of healthcare providers, which could include a primary care physician, a psychologist or psychiatrist, and a registered dietitian. Before starting any new treatment, always consult with these professionals. This combination of Modern medicine, Ayurveda, and Yoga should not replace conventional treatment but could potentially complement it.

ALLERGIC CONDITIONS

Allergies occur when the body's immune system reacts to a particular substance (allergen) as though it's harmful. Combining Modern medicine, Ayurveda, and Yoga can provide a holistic approach to manage allergies:

Modern Medicine Approaches

Antihistamines: These include medications like cetirizine, loratadine, and fexofenadine. They help to control the symptoms by blocking the effects of histamine, a substance in the body that causes allergic symptoms.

Corticosteroids: These may come in the form of nasal sprays, creams, or oral medications. They help to reduce inflammation and allergic reactions.

Immunotherapy: This involves exposure to gradually increasing amounts of the allergen to build up immunity.

Ayurvedic Approaches

In Ayurveda, allergies are often associated with a disturbance in the body's balance. Certain herbs and treatments can help to restore this balance:

Tulsi (Holy Basil): Known for its immune-boosting properties, it can help to combat allergens and reduce allergic reactions.

Turmeric (Curcuma longa): Its main component, curcumin, has anti-inflammatory and antioxidant properties.

Triphala: A traditional Ayurvedic formula that includes three fruits: Amalaki (Emblica officinalis), Bibhitaki (Terminalia bellirica), and Haritaki (Terminalia chebula). It supports the immune system and can help manage allergies.

Yogic Approaches

Yoga and Pranayama can support the immune system and help to calm the body, reducing allergic reactions:

Asanas: Poses like Fish Pose (Matsyasana), Cobra Pose (Bhujangasana), and Bridge Pose (Setu Bandhasana) can stimulate the thymus gland, boosting the immune system.

Pranayama: Breathing exercises like Kapalabhati and Nadi Shodhana (Alternate nostril breathing) can help to cleanse the body, improve circulation, and reduce allergic reactions.

Yogic Cleansing: Techniques such as Jal Neti (nasal irrigation with saline water) can help to clear the nasal passages, reducing symptoms of nasal allergies.

Synergy

Combining these approaches provides a comprehensive method for managing allergies:

Modern medications can provide quick relief from acute allergy symptoms.

Ayurvedic herbs and treatments can support the immune system and help to restore the body's balance, reducing allergic reactions.

Yoga and pranayama can support the immune system, improve circulation, and calm the body, reducing the severity and frequency of allergic reactions.

As always, the synergy of these treatments can be tailored to the individual's needs and provide a holistic approach to allergy management. Consult with a healthcare provider or knowledgeable practitioner to understand what treatment combination might work best.

ALZHEIMER's DESEASE

Alzheimer's disease is a progressive neurological disorder that impairs memory, thinking, and behaviour. The cause is unknown and there is currently no cure, but various treatments can help to manage the symptoms. A combined approach involving Modern medicine, Ayurveda, and Yoga can potentially provide comprehensive care:

Modern Medicine Approaches

Cholinesterase inhibitors: Drugs such as donepezil, rivastigmine, and galantamine are often used to treat the cognitive symptoms of Alzheimer's. They work by improving the levels of neurotransmitters in the brain.

Memantine: It works differently from cholinesterase inhibitors. It's used to improve memory, attention, reason, language and the ability to perform simple tasks.

Antidepressants, Anti-anxiety medications, Antipsychotics: These can be used to manage co-existing psychiatric symptoms such as depression, agitation or hallucinations.

Ayurvedic Approaches

In Ayurveda, Alzheimer's disease is often associated with the imbalance of Vata Dosha, specifically prana Vayu.

Brahmi (Bacopa monnieri): Known for its neuroprotective effects, it can help to improve memory and cognition.

Ashwagandha (Withania somnifera): Its neuroprotective properties may help to reduce stress and anxiety and protect the brain from degeneration.

Turmeric (Curcuma longa): The active component, curcumin, has anti-inflammatory and antioxidant properties and can potentially reduce cognitive decline.

Yogic Approaches

Yoga and meditation can support brain health, reduce stress, and improve cognitive function:

Asanas: Gentle yoga poses such as Tree Pose (Vrikshasana), Warrior III (Virabhadrasana III), and Corpse Pose (Shavasana) can help improve balance and coordination.

Pranayama: Breathing exercises like Anulom Vilom (Alternate Nostril Breathing) and Brahmari (Bee Breath) can help to calm the mind and improve focus.

Meditation: Mindfulness meditation and techniques such as Yoga Nidra (yogic sleep) can help to reduce stress and anxiety, improve mood, and support cognitive function.

Synergy

Modern medications can provide symptom relief and slow cognitive decline.

Ayurvedic herbs may provide neuroprotection, reduce inflammation, and help balance disturbed doshas.

Yoga and meditation can support mental well-being, reduce stress, and improve cognitive function.

This holistic approach could potentially enhance quality of life for patients with Alzheimer's. However, it's crucial that all treatments, particularly in the case of a serious condition like Alzheimer's, be overseen by a qualified healthcare provider. The use of these treatments should complement, not replace, conventional medical treatment.

PARKINSONISM

Parkinson's disease is a neurodegenerative disorder that affects movement control. It is characterized by symptoms such as tremors, stiffness, and difficulty with balance and coordination. A holistic approach involving Modern medicine, Ayurveda, and Yoga could potentially offer comprehensive care:

Modern Medicine Approaches

Levodopa: The most effective Parkinson's disease medication, usually combined with carbidopa.

Dopamine agonists: Medications like pramipexole and ropinirole, mimic the role of dopamine in the brain.

MAO B inhibitors: These include selegiline and rasagiline, which help prevent the breakdown of brain dopamine by inhibiting the brain enzyme monoamine oxidase B (MAO B).

Ayurvedic Approaches

In Ayurveda, Parkinson's disease (known as Kampavata) is attributed to Vata imbalance. Some Ayurvedic remedies include:

Ashwagandha (Withania somnifera): Known for its neuroprotective and anti-inflammatory properties, Ashwagandha may slow the progression of neurodegenerative diseases.

Brahmi (Bacopa monnieri): Used traditionally to enhance cognitive abilities, it might be beneficial in managing Parkinson's symptoms.

Zandopa: A herbal formulation of Mucuna pruriens (Velvet bean), which is a natural source of Levodopa.

Yogic Approaches

Yoga can help improve flexibility, balance, strength, and reduce stress in individuals with Parkinson's disease:

Asanas: Poses like Tadasana (Mountain Pose), Trikonasana (Triangle Pose), and Savasana (Corpse Pose) can help improve strength and balance.

Pranayama: Breathing techniques such as Anulom Vilom (Alternate Nostril Breathing) and Bhramari (Bee Breath) can help calm the mind.

Meditation: Techniques like mindfulness meditation can help manage stress and improve mental well-being.

Synergy

Modern medications can manage the symptoms and slow the progression of Parkinson's.

Ayurvedic treatments can provide additional neuroprotective effects and help to balance the Vata dosha.

Yoga can help manage the physical symptoms of Parkinson's and support mental well-being.

While this integrated approach has potential benefits, it's important that the implementation of these therapies be under the guidance of healthcare professionals, and the medications should always be taken as prescribed by a medical doctor.

SCIATICA

Sciatica is a condition characterized by pain going down the leg from the lower back, usually due to irritation of the sciatic nerve. This can be caused by conditions such as a herniated disc, spinal stenosis, or a pinched nerve. Here's how Modern medicine, Ayurveda, and Yoga can help manage sciatica:

Modern Medicine Approaches

Non-steroidal anti-inflammatory drugs (NSAIDs): Drugs such as ibuprofen can help reduce inflammation and pain.

Muscle relaxants: Medications like cyclobenzaprine can help relieve muscle spasms.

Corticosteroids: Oral or injected steroids can help reduce inflammation and pain.

Physical Therapy: Guided exercises can help strengthen muscles and improve posture and flexibility.

Ayurvedic Approaches

In Ayurveda, sciatica (known as Gridhrasi) is usually associated with an imbalance of Vata dosha.

Ashwagandha (Withania somnifera): Known for its anti-inflammatory properties, it may help reduce nerve irritation.

Ginkgo Biloba and Coenzyme Q – Effective in reducing the nerve pain and providing nerve strength. Its also available with beet Root Extract and Green Tea extract in form of Super Nerve Power that also has phosphodiesterase inhibitor to add strength to pain reduction and neuromodulation.

Guggulu (Commiphora mukul): It has anti-inflammatory and analgesic properties, which can help reduce inflammation and relieve pain.

Rasna (Pluchea lanceolata): It is often used for its analgesic and anti-inflammatory properties in Ayurvedic treatments for sciatica.

Yogic Approaches

Yoga can help stretch and strengthen muscles, improve posture, and reduce pain:

Asanas: Gentle backbends, twists, and hamstring stretches can help relieve pressure on the sciatic nerve. Poses like Sphinx Pose, Supine Twist, and Reclining Hand-to-Big-Toe Pose can be beneficial.

Pranayama: Breathing exercises like Dirga Pranayama (Three-Part Breath) and Ujjayi Pranayama (Victorious Breath) can help relax the body and mind.

Synergy

Modern medications can provide immediate pain relief and reduce inflammation.

Ayurvedic herbs may help further reduce inflammation and help correct the underlying dosha imbalance.

Yoga can help stretch and strengthen muscles, improve flexibility and posture, and reduce future instances of sciatica.

This integrated approach may provide a comprehensive way to manage sciatica. However, the treatment should be guided by healthcare professionals, and the implementation of any new treatment, especially in the case of serious conditions like sciatica, should always be discussed with a healthcare provider.

PROSTATIC HYPERTROPHY

Benign prostatic hyperplasia (BPH), also known as prostatic hypertrophy, is a common condition as men get older. It's caused by an enlargement of the prostate gland, which can lead to urinary symptoms. Here's how Modern medicine, Ayurveda, and Yoga can help manage BPH:

Modern Medicine Approaches

Alpha blockers: Medications such as tamsulosin and alfuzosin can help relax the muscles of the prostate and bladder neck, improving urine flow.

5-Alpha reductase inhibitors: Drugs like finasteride and dutasteride can help shrink the prostate by reducing levels of a hormone that makes it grow.

Phosphodiesterase-5 Inhibitors: Medications like tadalafil can also be used to improve symptoms of BPH.

Ayurvedic Approaches

In Ayurveda, BPH is seen as an imbalance in the Pitta and Vata doshas.

Varuna (Crataeva nurvala): This herb is used for urinary disorders and can help improve urinary symptoms.

Gokshura (Tribulus terrestris): Known to improve urinary tract health and has anti-inflammatory properties.

Shilajit: A resin with anti-inflammatory properties that can potentially help shrink the prostate.

Yogic Approaches

Yoga can help improve the overall functioning of the body and reduce symptoms:

Asanas: Certain poses such as Baddha Konasana (Bound Angle Pose), Bhujangasana (Cobra Pose), and Janu Sirsasana (Head-to-Knee Pose) can improve pelvic floor health and urinary function.

Pranayama: Deep breathing exercises such as Kapalabhati (Skull Shining Breath) and Anulom Vilom (Alternate Nostril Breathing) can reduce stress and improve overall health.

Synergy

Modern medications can directly target symptoms and the cause of BPH, reducing prostate size and improving urinary function.

Ayurvedic herbs can provide additional symptomatic relief and potentially help to balance the underlying dosha imbalances.

Yoga can contribute to overall health and wellness, reduce stress, and help manage BPH symptoms.

It's important to note that these treatments should be guided by healthcare professionals, and the medications should always be taken as prescribed by a medical doctor. Additionally, while Ayurvedic and Yoga therapies can support Modern treatments, they should not replace them.

RECURRENT URINARY INFECTIONS

Recurrent urinary tract infections (UTIs) can be a challenging condition to manage. They are most commonly caused by bacteria that enter the urethra and then the bladder. Here's how Modern medicine, Ayurveda, and Yoga can help manage recurrent UTIs:

Modern Medicine Approaches

Antibiotics: The most common treatment for UTIs are antibiotics such as Nitrofurantoin, Fosfomycin, or Trimethoprim/sulfamethoxazole. These can be used for both acute treatment and prophylaxis.

Pain relief: Phenazopyridine is a medication that can alleviate discomfort or pain during urination.

Topical estrogen: For post-menopausal women, topical estrogen can help prevent UTIs by changing the flora of the vagina.

Ayurvedic Approaches

In Ayurveda, UTIs are often linked to an imbalance in Pitta dosha, which governs heat and metabolism in the body.

Cumin (Jeera): Its cooling property can help in balancing the Pitta dosha and its diuretic property can help flush out the bacteria causing the infection.

Gokshura (Tribulus terrestris): Known for its diuretic properties, it can help promote urinary health.

Coriander (Dhania): Its cooling properties can help balance Pitta dosha and also promote urinary health.

Yogic Approaches

Yoga can support the immune system, reduce stress, and improve the health of the urinary system:

Asanas: Poses that stimulate the urinary bladder like Bhujangasana (Cobra Pose), Ardha Matsyendrasana (Half Lord of the Fishes Pose), and Pawanmuktasana (Wind Relieving Pose) may help.

Pranayama: Breathing exercises like Kapalbhati (Skull Shining Breath) and Anulom Vilom (Alternate Nostril Breathing) can help improve immunity and reduce stress.

Synergy

Modern medications provide the first line of defense, offering direct antibacterial activity against the UTI.

Ayurvedic herbs support this, offering further antibacterial, anti-inflammatory, and diuretic effects. They also help balance the underlying dosha imbalance, especially if it's a Pitta disorder.

Yoga supports overall health, strengthening the immune system, reducing stress, and helping improve the health of the urinary system.

As always, it's important to consult with healthcare professionals before starting or changing any treatments. Any new treatment should be discussed with a healthcare provider to ensure it's safe and suitable for the individual's circumstances.

SEBORRHOEA

Seborrhoeic dermatitis, also known as seborrhoea, is a common skin disease that mainly affects your scalp. It causes scaly patches, red skin, and stubborn dandruff. It can also affect oily areas of the body, like the face, sides of the nose, eyebrows, ears, eyelids, and chest. Here's how Modern medicine, Ayurveda, and Yoga can help manage seborrhoea:

Modern Medicine Approaches

Antifungal Medications: Topical antifungals like ketoconazole, or ciclopirox can help control the yeast growth that often worsens seborrhea. Antifungal shapoo are also used and some times help.

Topical Steroids: These can help reduce inflammation and control flare-ups, but they should not be used long term. Examples include hydrocortisone and fluocinolone.

Coal Tar: Products with coal tar may help slow skin cell growth and improve seborrhoea.

Ayurvedic Approaches

Ayurveda sees seborrhea as an imbalance of Kapha and Vata doshas.

Neem (Azadirachta indica): Known for its anti-inflammatory and antifungal properties, Neem can help manage symptoms of seborrhoea when applied topically.

Turmeric (Curcuma longa): Turmeric's anti-inflammatory properties can help reduce the redness and inflammation associated with seborrhoea.

Aloe Vera: Applying Aloe Vera gel can help soothe the skin and reduce inflammation and itchiness.

Yogic Approaches

Yoga can help improve the overall functioning of the body and reduce stress, which can trigger or worsen seborrhoea:

Asanas: Postures that promote blood circulation to the head like Adho Mukha Svanasana (Downward-Facing Dog) and Sirsasana (Headstand) may be beneficial.

Pranayama: Breathing exercises like Kapalbhati (Skull Shining Breath) and Anulom Vilom (Alternate Nostril Breathing) can help reduce stress and improve overall health.

Synergy

Modern medications can directly target symptoms of seborrhea, providing immediate relief and controlling flare-ups.

Ayurvedic herbs can provide additional symptomatic relief and can help to balance the underlying dosha imbalances.

Yoga can contribute to overall health and wellness, reduce stress, and potentially help manage seborrhea symptoms.

As always, the adoption of these practices should be guided by healthcare professionals. The medications should always be taken as prescribed by a medical doctor. Moreover, while Ayurvedic and Yoga therapies can support Modern treatments, they should not replace them. They can serve as a part of a comprehensive approach to managing seborrhoea.

NEPHROTIC SYNDROME

Nephrotic syndrome is a kidney disorder that causes your body to excrete too much protein in your urine, leading to swelling in different parts of the body. It's crucial to consult a healthcare provider for an appropriate treatment plan as this is a serious condition. Here's how Modern medicine, Ayurveda, and Yoga can help manage nephrotic syndrome:

Modern Medicine Approaches

Corticosteroids: Prednisone is a common treatment for nephrotic syndrome to reduce inflammation and the immune response.

Immunosuppressive Drugs: Medications such as cyclosporine and rituximab may be used to regulate the immune system and decrease the body's reaction.

ACE inhibitors and ARBs: These medications, such as lisinopril and losartan, can reduce protein loss and control blood pressure.

Ayurvedic Approaches

In Ayurveda, nephrotic syndrome might be correlated with conditions caused by an imbalance in all three doshas, though primarily Kapha.

Punarnava (Boerhavia diffusa): This herb is known for its diuretic and anti-inflammatory properties, which can help manage swelling and kidney function.

Gokshura (Tribulus terrestris): Known for its diuretic properties and its potential ability to support kidney function.

Varuna (Crataeva nurvala): This herb is traditionally used for urinary and kidney disorders and might aid in managing symptoms of nephrotic syndrome.

Yogic Approaches

Yoga can support overall wellbeing and stress reduction, which is essential for managing chronic diseases:

Asanas: Gentle poses that promote blood flow to the kidneys such as Paschimottanasana (Seated Forward Bend) and Setu Bandhasana (Bridge Pose) may be beneficial.

Pranayama: Breathing exercises such as Anulom Vilom (Alternate Nostril Breathing) and Bhramari Pranayama (Humming Bee Breath) can help in stress reduction.

Synergy

Modern medicine provides direct treatment, targeting the kidney inflammation and regulating the immune response with corticosteroids and immunosuppressive drugs.

Ayurvedic herbs can help manage symptoms, support kidney function, and balance the body's overall energy (doshas).

Yoga can promote overall health, strengthen the immune system, reduce stress, and help manage symptoms.

It's essential to consult healthcare professionals before starting or changing treatments. All these treatments should be used in coordination and under the guidance of appropriate medical professionals.

ACNE

Acne is a common skin condition that occurs when your hair follicles become plugged with oil and dead skin cells. It often causes whiteheads, blackheads, or pimples, usually on the face, forehead, chest, upper back, and shoulders. Let's look at how Modern medicine, Ayurveda, and Yoga can help manage acne:

Modern Medicine Approaches

Topical Retinoids: Medications such as adapalene, tretinoin, and tazarotene help to prevent plugging of follicles.

Antibiotics: Topical or oral antibiotics, like clindamycin or doxycycline, can help fight bacterial infection and reduce inflammation.

Oral Contraceptives: For women, certain types of oral contraceptives can help regulate hormone levels and reduce acne.

Ayurvedic Approaches

In Ayurveda, acne is typically considered an imbalance of the Pitta dosha.

Neem (Azadirachta indica): Neem has antibacterial properties that can help fight acne-causing bacteria when applied topically.

Turmeric (Curcuma longa): Turmeric has anti-inflammatory properties that can reduce redness and inflammation from acne.

Aloe Vera: Applying Aloe Vera gel can help soothe the skin, reduce inflammation, and aid in healing.

Yogic Approaches

Yoga can help by reducing stress levels, improving circulation, and detoxifying the body:

Asanas: Poses like the Cobra Pose (Bhujangasana), Bow Pose (Dhanurasana), and Fish Pose (Matsyasana) stimulate the digestive system and help detoxify the body.

Pranayama: Breathing exercises like Kapalbhati (Skull Shining Breath) and Anulom Vilom (Alternate Nostril Breathing) help reduce stress and detoxify the body.

Synergy

Modern medications can directly target the symptoms of acne, providing immediate relief and preventing future breakouts.

Ayurvedic herbs can provide additional symptomatic relief, aid in healing, and help to balance the underlying dosha imbalance.

Yoga can improve overall health, reduce stress (a common trigger for acne), and help detoxify the body, which may help in managing acne symptoms.

As always, these practices should be guided by healthcare professionals. Medications should always be taken as prescribed by a medical doctor, and while Ayurvedic and Yoga therapies can support Modern treatments, they should not replace them. They can serve as part of a comprehensive approach to managing acne.

EYE SIGHT PROBLEMS

Eye health and vision problems can be managed through a combination of Modern medicine, Ayurveda, and Yoga. Below, I'll provide an overview of potential solutions in each of these fields. Please note that these should not be seen as comprehensive treatment plans but as potential components of a larger approach, under the guidance of a medical professional.

Modern Medicine Approaches

For eyesight problems, the exact treatment will depend on the specific condition. Here are some general approaches:

Corrective Lenses: Glasses or contact lenses are commonly used to correct refractive errors such as myopia (short-sightedness), hypermetropia (long-sightedness), and astigmatism.

Medications: Eye drops or oral medications may be prescribed for conditions like glaucoma, dry eye syndrome, or infections.

Surgery: For some conditions, such as cataracts or severe refractive errors, surgery may be recommended.

Ayurvedic Approaches

Ayurveda offers several methods for maintaining eye health and treating eye conditions, considering it a Pitta domain:

Triphala: A combination of Amalaki (Emblica officinalis), Bibhitaki (Terminalia bellirica), and Haritaki (Terminalia chebula) is often used to support eye health. It's rich in antioxidants and believed to support the health of eye tissues.

Amalaki (Emblica officinalis): Also known as Indian Gooseberry, Amalaki is high in Vitamin C and antioxidants, which may be beneficial for overall eye health.

Yashtimadhu (Glycyrrhiza glabra): Yashtimadhu is believed to be helpful in treating various eye diseases due to its anti-inflammatory properties.

Yogic Approaches

Certain yoga exercises and pranayama can help in enhancing eye health:

Eye Yoga Exercises: Specific movements, like looking up and down, side to side, or rotating the eyes in circles, can help strengthen the eye muscles and maintain eye health.

Tratak Meditation: This meditation involves focusing the eyes and mind on a single point, often a candle flame, without blinking. This exercise may help to improve focus and concentration.

Pranayama: Breathing exercises, like Anulom Vilom (Alternate Nostril Breathing) and Kapalbhati (Skull Shining Breath), can help increase the oxygen supply to the eyes and the brain, which may help maintain eye health.

Synergy

Modern medicine provides immediate and targeted intervention for specific eye conditions, such as refractive errors, glaucoma, and cataracts.

Ayurvedic herbs can help manage symptoms and support the overall health of eye tissues.

Yogic exercises can help strengthen eye muscles, improve focus, and provide relaxation, reducing stress that could impact eye health.

All these treatments should be used in coordination and under the guidance of appropriate medical professionals. Eye conditions can be serious, and any changes in vision should be evaluated by a healthcare professional promptly.

HEART FAILURE

The management of heart failure involves a multi-faceted approach that includes Modern medicine, lifestyle changes, and potentially complementary therapies such as Yoga and Ayurveda. It is critical to note that all of these suggestions should be discussed with and monitored by healthcare professionals, as heart failure is a serious condition.

Modern Medicine Approaches

ACE inhibitors (Angiotensin-converting enzyme inhibitors) such as Enalapril, Lisinopril, or Ramipril are often used to lower blood pressure and reduce strain on the heart.

Beta-blockers like Metoprolol, Carvedilol, and Bisoprolol are used to slow the heart rate and reduce blood pressure, again reducing strain on the heart.

Diuretics (water pills) such as Furosemide (Lasix) or Bumetanide can help reduce fluid buildup in the body, a common symptom of heart failure.

Aldosterone antagonists like Spironolactone and Eplerenone can help people with severe heart failure symptoms.

ARBs (Angiotensin II Receptor Blockers) and ARNIs (Angiotensin Receptor-Neprilysin Inhibitors) may also be prescribed.

Ayurvedic Approaches

Arjuna (Terminalia Arjuna): Arjuna is a herb well-regarded in Ayurvedic medicine for heart conditions due to its antioxidant and anti-inflammatory properties.

Punarnava (Boerhavia diffusa): This herb is used in Ayurveda for its diuretic properties, which may help with fluid retention, a common issue in heart failure.

Hridayarnava Rasa: An Ayurvedic mineral formulation used in the treatment of cardiac disorders.

Yogic Approaches

Gentle Yoga Asanas: Gentle movement can be beneficial, but it's important not to overexert oneself. Poses such as the Legs-Up-The-Wall Pose (Viparita Karani) can be calming and might help reduce symptoms like edema.

Pranayama: Controlled breathing exercises, like Anulom Vilom (Alternate Nostril Breathing), can aid in reducing stress and promoting relaxation.

Meditation: Mindfulness and meditation can help manage the stress and emotional challenges associated with managing a chronic illness like heart failure.

Synergy

Modern medicine offers targeted medications to manage the symptoms of heart failure and reduce the workload of the heart.

Ayurveda may provide supportive therapies to manage symptoms, support overall heart health, and reduce side effects from other treatments. It's important to discuss these with your doctor, especially due to potential interactions with other medications.

Yoga, specifically gentle poses and breathing exercises, can help manage stress, promote relaxation, and increase overall well-being.

Remember, it is crucial to discuss any changes to medication, or any addition of Ayurvedic or yogic practices, with the healthcare team managing heart failure. This ensures a safe, integrated, and holistic approach to managing the condition.

HEPATITIS

Managing hepatitis requires a comprehensive approach, which could potentially involve Modern medicine, Ayurveda, and Yoga. It's important to note that all of these suggestions should be discussed with and monitored by healthcare professionals, as hepatitis is a serious condition.

Modern Medicine Approaches

Antiviral Medications: Depending on the type of hepatitis, antiviral medications like Entecavir, Tenofovir, or Sofosbuvir may be prescribed.

Immunosuppressive Medication: In some cases, like autoimmune hepatitis, drugs that suppress the immune system like Prednisone or Azathioprine might be used.

Liver Protectants: Medications like Silymarin (milk thistle) may be used to support liver health.

Ayurvedic Approaches

Bhumyamalaki (Phyllanthus niruri): This herb is traditionally used in Ayurveda for liver conditions, including hepatitis, due to its hepatoprotective and antiviral properties.

Kalmegh (Andrographis paniculata): Kalmegh is another Ayurvedic herb often used for liver conditions because of its hepatoprotective properties.

Arogyavardhini Vati: This is a herbal-mineral formulation used in Ayurveda that's often recommended for liver conditions.

Yogic Approaches

Gentle Yoga Asanas: Gentle yoga asanas, particularly those that stimulate the liver area, can be beneficial. Poses such as the Cobra Pose (Bhujangasana), Bow Pose (Dhanurasana), and Spinal Twist (Ardha Matsyendrasana) may be useful.

Pranayama: Breathing exercises like Kapalabhati and Anulom Vilom (Alternate Nostril Breathing) can be helpful. However, Kapalabhati should be performed under supervision and might not be suitable for everyone.

Meditation: Meditation techniques can help manage the stress associated with chronic diseases like hepatitis.

Synergy

Modern medicines aim to control the viral load, alleviate symptoms, and prevent progression of the disease.

Ayurvedic herbs and formulations might offer supportive therapies to improve liver function and mitigate symptoms. It's important to discuss these with your doctor, especially due to potential interactions with other medications.

Yoga can help manage stress, promote relaxation, and support overall well-being. The poses can improve digestion and circulation to the liver, supporting its detoxification processes.

Remember, it is crucial to discuss any changes to medication or any addition of Ayurvedic or yogic practices with the healthcare team managing hepatitis. This ensures a safe and integrated approach to managing the condition.

AUTISM

Autism Spectrum Disorder (ASD) is a neurodevelopmental disorder characterized by difficulties with social interaction, communication, and repetitive or restrictive behaviors. It's essential to understand that no single approach is 'the best,' and each individual's unique needs should be considered. Here's how Modern medicine, Ayurveda, and yoga might be helpful in managing ASD:

Modern Medicine Approaches

Behavioral Therapy: Applied Behavior Analysis (ABA) is a type of therapy used to improve specific behaviors in individuals with autism. It's considered the "gold standard" treatment.

Medications: Certain medications, like Risperidone or Aripiprazole, can be used to manage associated symptoms such as aggression, hyperactivity, or self-injurious behavior.

Ayurvedic Approaches

Medhya Rasayanas: These are group of herbs known to improve mental capabilities. Brahmi (Bacopa monnieri), Mandukaparni (Centella asiatica), Shankhapushpi (Convolvulus pluricaulis) and Jatamansi (Nardostachys jatamansi) are examples.

Panchakarma: Ayurvedic detoxification therapies like Panchakarma can be helpful in balancing the doshas and improving overall health.

Yogic Approaches

Asanas: Yoga postures such as the Tree Pose (Vrikshasana), Warrior Pose (Virabhadrasana), and Child's Pose (Balasana) can help improve balance, coordination, and body awareness.

Pranayama: Breathing exercises, especially Anulom Vilom (Alternate Nostril Breathing) and Bhramari (Humming Bee Breath), can promote relaxation and help manage anxiety.

Yoga Nidra: A deep relaxation technique can help in managing stress and anxiety, common in individuals with autism.

Synergy

Modern medications and behavioral therapies can manage associated behavioral challenges and improve communication and social skills.

Ayurvedic herbs could potentially support cognitive function and overall well-being, while Panchakarma may improve general health and well-being. It's crucial to discuss these with a healthcare provider.

Yoga, especially when tailored for the individual, can provide a non-competitive, calming environment for physical activity. It can also support stress management, body awareness, and motor skills.

It's crucial to understand that these are potential strategies, and the effectiveness can vary greatly among individuals. Therefore, all treatments and approaches should be discussed with a healthcare provider to ensure they are suitable for the individual's unique needs. Also, it's important to note that these treatments are to support the individual with autism and not to 'cure' autism, as autism is a part of the individual's unique identity.

OSTEOPOROSIS

Osteoporosis is a condition characterized by a decrease in bone density, making bones fragile and more susceptible to fractures. The integration of Modern medicine, Ayurveda, and Yoga can form a comprehensive approach for managing osteoporosis:

Modern Medicine Approaches

Medications: Bisphosphonates (e.g., Alendronate, Risedronate), Calcitonin, and Denosumab are often prescribed to slow bone loss. In some cases, Teriparatide, Abaloparatide, or Romosozumab may be used to stimulate bone growth.

Supplements: Adequate calcium and Vitamin D intake is essential for bone health. Depending on diet and sunlight exposure, supplements may be necessary.

Ayurvedic Approaches

Herbs and Minerals: Herbs like Hadjod (Cissus quadrangularis) and Ashwagandha (Withania somnifera), and minerals like Praval Pishti (coral calcium) are believed to enhance bone health.

Balancing Vata: Osteoporosis is considered a Vata disorder in Ayurveda, so therapies (like oil massage or Abhyanga) aimed at balancing Vata could be beneficial.

Yogic Approaches

Asanas: Weight-bearing poses like Tadasana (Mountain Pose), Virabhadrasana (Warrior Pose), Trikonasana (Triangle Pose), and Setu Bandhasana (Bridge Pose) can improve bone strength.

Pranayama: Practices such as Kapalbhati (Skull Shining Breath) and Anulom Vilom (Alternate Nostril Breathing) can help maintain overall health and reduce stress.

Synergy

Modern medications and supplements can directly target the underlying issue of bone loss.

Ayurvedic herbs may provide a natural support for bone health, while Vata balancing therapies could improve overall wellbeing. Always discuss the use of herbs with a healthcare provider.

Yoga asanas, especially weight-bearing ones, could potentially slow bone loss and improve balance, reducing the risk of falls and fractures. Pranayama practices can enhance overall health and wellbeing.

A combined approach offers an overall strategy for managing osteoporosis by directly addressing bone health, promoting overall wellbeing, and potentially reducing the risk of fractures. As always, it's important to discuss any new therapies with a healthcare provider to ensure they are safe and suitable for the individual's condition.

DRUG ADDICTION

Managing drug addiction is a very complex process that often involves a combination of medical, psychological, and lifestyle approaches. There is no single approach that will work for all as different drugs have different addiction potential and approaches and different personalities and co-morbidies make it even more complex. Here is a simplistic approach how Modern medicine, Ayurveda, and Yoga can all play integral roles in the recovery process:

Modern Medicine Approaches

Medications: Depending on the specific substance of addiction, various medications can be used to manage withdrawal symptoms and reduce cravings. For opioid addiction, Methadone, Buprenorphine, and Naltrexone are often used. Disulfiram, Naltrexone, and Acamprosate might be used for alcohol addiction.

Psychotherapy: Cognitive-behavioral therapy, contingency management, motivational enhancement therapy, and 12-step facilitation are commonly utilized psychological approaches for managing drug addiction.

Ayurvedic Approaches

Herbs: Ashwagandha (Withania somnifera), Brahmi (Bacopa monnieri), and Jatamansi (Nardostachys jatamansi) are commonly used in Ayurveda for their potential to reduce anxiety, improve mental clarity, and support overall brain health.

Panchakarma: This is a detoxifying process in Ayurveda that can help cleanse the body of toxins and rebalance the doshas.

Yogic Approaches

Asanas: Yoga postures, such as Balasana (Child's Pose), Savasana (Corpse Pose), and various inversion poses, can help reduce anxiety and promote relaxation.

Pranayama: Breathing techniques such as Anulom Vilom (Alternate Nostril Breathing) and Bhramari Pranayama (Bee Breathing) can help calm the mind.

Meditation and Mindfulness: Regular practice can enhance self-control, increase self-awareness, and reduce cravings.

Synergy

Modern medications can help manage withdrawal symptoms and reduce cravings, making the recovery process more manageable.

Ayurvedic herbs and Panchakarma may support the body's healing process and improve overall well-being.

Yoga can provide a valuable set of tools for managing stress, improving mental health, and enhancing self-awareness, all of which are critical in the recovery process.

The integrated approach could help a person dealing with drug addiction navigate their recovery more successfully by targeting physical symptoms, supporting overall health, and providing tools for stress management and mental health care. It's crucial that anyone attempting to overcome addiction does so under the supervision of healthcare professionals.

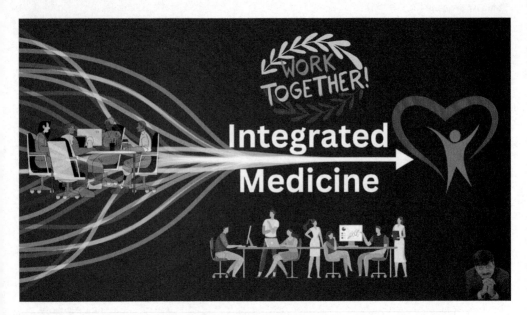

Synopsis of Integrative Approach to Health Conditions Using Modern Medicine, Ayurveda, and Yoga

The holistic treatment of various health conditions can be effectively managed using a synergistic approach that incorporates modern medicine, Ayurveda, and yoga. These diverse practices offer different yet complementary strategies that enhance patient care when used together.

1. Diabetes

Modern medicine utilizes insulin and oral hypoglycemic agents to manage diabetes. Ayurveda provides lifestyle and diet modifications along with herbal remedies such as Gymnema sylvestre. Yoga asanas and pranayama, such as Vrikshasana and Anulom Vilom, help in reducing stress levels and improving metabolism, contributing to better glucose control.

2. Hypertension

Antihypertensive medications like ACE inhibitors and beta-blockers are used in conventional medicine. Ayurvedic herbs like Arjuna (Terminalia arjuna) and diet changes can also support heart health. Yoga techniques such as the Corpse Pose (Savasana) and breathing exercises help manage stress, a major contributing factor to hypertension.

3. Chronic Arthritis

Western medicine uses NSAIDs and DMARDs for pain management and disease progression. Ayurveda suggests herbs like Nirgundi (Vitex negundo) and Ashwagandha (Withania somnifera) and Panchakarma therapy. Gentle yoga exercises like Sukhasana (Easy Pose) help improve joint flexibility.

4. Dementia

Cholinesterase inhibitors are typically used in modern medicine for dementia. Ayurveda recommends Brahmi (Bacopa monnieri) for cognitive enhancement. Yoga and meditation can help improve memory and cognitive function, and reduce stress.

5. Chronic Asthma

Western medicine employs bronchodilators and corticosteroids for asthma. Ayurveda uses herbal preparations like Sitopaladi Churna, and yoga provides beneficial practices like Pranayama for better breath control.

6. Migraine

Pain relievers and triptans are used in conventional medicine for migraines. Ayurveda suggests herbs like Jatamansi (Nardostachys jatamansi) and yoga techniques like Balasana (Child's Pose) help in managing stress and reducing migraine intensity.

7. Irritable Bowel Syndrome

Antispasmodic and anti-diarrheal medications are used in conventional medicine. Ayurveda suggests herbal medicines like Kutaj (Holarrhena antidysenterica) and yoga postures like Pavanamuktasana (Wind-Relieving Pose) for better digestion.

8. Obesity

Modern medicine uses medications, behavioral therapy, and surgical interventions. Ayurveda offers herbs like Guggul (Commiphora mukul) and a dietary regimen. Yoga practices like Surya Namaskar (Sun Salutation) support weight loss.

9. Depression

Antidepressants, psychotherapy, and cognitive-behavioral therapy are conventional methods. Ayurveda suggests herbs like Ashwagandha (Withania somnifera). Yoga and meditation provide stress relief and mood enhancement.

10. Drug Addiction

Western medicines help manage withdrawal symptoms and reduce cravings. Ayurveda uses herbs like Ashwagandha (Withania somnifera) and Panchakarma for detoxification. Yoga, especially meditation, enhances self-control and reduces cravings.

This synopsis shows how modern medicine, Ayurveda, and yoga can be used collectively for a more holistic approach to healthcare. The combination of these methods may help improve treatment outcomes and enhance the overall quality of life for patients with various conditions. Always consult with healthcare professionals for personalized treatment plans.

11. Chronic Eczema

Modern medicine employs corticosteroids and other medications to reduce inflammation and itching. Ayurvedic treatments such as applying Neem (Azadirachta indica) oil can also be beneficial. Yoga, specifically practices like Bhujangasana (Cobra Pose), may help reduce stress which can exacerbate eczema.

12. Dysmenorrhoea

Non-steroidal anti-inflammatory drugs (NSAIDs) are commonly used in western medicine to relieve menstrual pain. Ayurveda may recommend herbs like Ashoka (Saraca asoca) and Shatavari (Asparagus racemosus). Specific yoga asanas, such as the Butterfly Pose (Baddha Konasana), can help alleviate menstrual discomfort.

13. Chronic Fatigue Syndrome

While there is no specific treatment for this in conventional medicine, management strategies involve treating symptoms such as pain and sleep problems. Ayurveda employs Ashwagandha (Withania somnifera) to boost energy. Yoga practices like Balasana (Child's Pose) may offer relaxation and energy conservation.

14. Systemic Lupus Erythematosus (SLE)

Modern medicine uses NSAIDs, corticosteroids, and immunosuppressants to manage SLE. Ayurveda uses herbs such as Guduchi (Tinospora cordifolia) to modulate the immune system. Yoga asanas like the Fish Pose (Matsyasana) help in reducing stress and promoting physical flexibility.

15. Multiple Sclerosis

While modern medicine may use corticosteroids and physical therapy to manage symptoms, Ayurveda utilizes Ashwagandha (Withania somnifera) to strengthen the nervous system. Yoga practices such as Tadasana (Mountain Pose) may help improve balance and coordination.

16. Fibromyalgia

Conventional treatments include pain relievers, antidepressants, and anti-seizure drugs. Ayurveda suggests using Dashmool (a combination of 10 roots) for its analgesic properties. Restorative yoga poses such as Savasana (Corpse Pose) can help manage pain and fatigue.

17. Hypothyroidism

In modern medicine, synthetic thyroid hormone is used. Ayurveda employs Guggul (Commiphora mukul) for its potential to improve thyroid function. Asanas like Sarvangasana (Shoulder Stand) might stimulate the thyroid gland.

18. Hyperthyroidism

Anti-thyroid medications and radioactive iodine are common treatments. Ayurvedic herbs such as Bugleweed (Lycopus europaeus) might help regulate thyroid hormone levels. Pranayama techniques, like Kapalbhati, could also aid in hormonal balance.

19. Anxiety Disorder

Antidepressants, sedatives, and psychotherapy are used in conventional treatments. Ayurvedic herbs such as Brahmi (Bacopa monnieri) can reduce anxiety. Yoga and meditation practices are powerful tools for managing stress and promoting relaxation.

These examples highlight the powerful potential of a synergistic approach that integrates modern medicine, Ayurveda, and yoga for a holistic treatment strategy. Always consult with healthcare professionals for personalized treatment plans.

20. Depression

Antidepressants and psychotherapy form the primary treatment strategy in modern medicine. Ayurveda uses herbs like Brahmi (Bacopa monnieri) for its calming effect. Regular practice of yoga and meditation may promote mindfulness and alleviate symptoms of depression.

21. Attention Deficit Hyperactivity Disorder (ADHD)

Stimulant medications and behavior therapy are the mainstay of conventional treatment. Ayurveda uses Brahmi (Bacopa monnieri) to enhance brain function. Yoga postures and breathing exercises can improve focus and decrease hyperactivity.

22. Insomnia

Sleeping pills and behavior therapies are common in western medicine. Ayurveda suggests using herbs like Ashwagandha (Withania somnifera) to promote sleep. Yoga Nidra and certain Pranayama techniques may promote deep rest and better sleep patterns.

23. Anorexia Nervosa

Modern medicine combines nutritional therapy with psychological therapy. Ayurvedic treatments may include the use of herbs like Ashwagandha (Withania somnifera) for its nourishing properties. Yoga and meditation may be beneficial for managing stress and promoting body positivity.

24. Allergy

Antihistamines and corticosteroids form the mainstay of modern allergy treatment. Ayurveda uses herbs like Haridra (Curcuma longa) for its anti-inflammatory and antihistaminic properties. Breathing exercises like Anulom Vilom Pranayama may aid in managing respiratory allergies.

25. Alzheimer's Disease

Cholinesterase inhibitors and memantine are commonly used in western medicine. Ayurvedic herbs like Brahmi (Bacopa monnieri) can enhance cognitive function. Yoga and meditation can help improve mental agility and memory.

26. Parkinson's Disease

Dopaminergic medications are used in modern medicine. Ayurveda may suggest the use of Mucuna pruriens, which contains natural levodopa. Yoga may aid in maintaining mobility and balance.

27. Sciatica

Pain relievers and physiotherapy are common treatments. Ayurveda uses herbs like Guggul (Commiphora mukul) for its anti-inflammatory properties. Gentle yoga postures such as Ardha Matsyendrasana (Half Spinal Twist) may help to stretch and strengthen the back muscles.

28. Prostatic Hypertrophy

Medications to shrink the prostate or relax muscles are used in modern medicine. Ayurveda uses herbs like Varuna (Crataeva nurvala) for its potential effects on prostate health. Yoga practices such as the Forward Bending Pose (Pashchimottanasana) can promote pelvic health.

29. Recurrent Urinary Infections

Antibiotics are the primary treatment in western medicine. Ayurveda uses herbs like Gokshura (Tribulus terrestris) for its diuretic and antimicrobial properties. Yoga asanas such as Bhadrasana (Butterfly Pose) can help promote urinary health.

30. Seborrhoea

Topical creams and shampoos form the mainstay of treatment. Ayurveda employs Neem (Azadirachta indica) for its antifungal properties. Yoga poses that increase blood circulation to the head like Adho Mukha Svanasana (Downward-Facing Dog) can help improve scalp health.

These examples highlight the powerful potential of a synergistic approach that integrates modern medicine, Ayurveda, and yoga for a holistic treatment strategy. Always consult with healthcare professionals for personalized treatment plans.

31. Nephrotic Syndrome

Western treatment usually involves corticosteroids, diuretics, and angiotensin-converting enzyme (ACE) inhibitors. Ayurveda might use Gokshura (Tribulus terrestris) for its diuretic and kidney protective properties. Certain yoga poses like Setu Bandhasana (Bridge Pose) can help improve kidney function.

32. Acne

Modern medicine treats acne with topical retinoids, antibiotics, and sometimes hormonal therapies. Ayurveda recommends Neem (Azadirachta indica) and Turmeric (Curcuma longa) for their antimicrobial and anti-inflammatory properties. Facial yoga exercises can improve blood circulation to the face, promoting healthier skin.

33. Eye Sight Problems

Corrective glasses, contact lenses, or surgical procedures are the main western medical treatments. Ayurveda suggests Triphala for its potential eye health benefits. Tratak (candle gazing) and certain eye exercises in yoga can help strengthen eye muscles.

34. Heart Failure

Diuretics, beta-blockers, and ACE inhibitors are used in western medicine. Arjuna (Terminalia arjuna) is used in Ayurveda for its potential cardiovascular benefits. Yoga practices like gentle Pranayama can help improve heart health.

35. Hepatitis

Modern medicine uses antiviral medications and vaccines for treatment. Ayurveda employs herbs like Bhumyamalaki (Phyllanthus niruri) for its antiviral properties. Gentle yoga asanas and Pranayama can enhance overall liver health.

36. Autism

Therapy and medication to manage symptoms are the primary western medical treatments. Ayurveda uses herbs like Brahmi (Bacopa monnieri) to improve cognitive function. Yoga and meditation can enhance self-awareness and social interaction skills.

37. Osteoporosis

Western medicine uses bisphosphonates and hormone replacement therapy. Ayurveda recommends herbs like Hadjod (Cissus quadrangularis) for its potential bone-healing properties. Weight-bearing yoga asanas like Tadasana (Mountain Pose) can help improve bone density.

38. Drug Addiction

Modern medicine uses detoxification, counseling, and medications to treat addiction. Ayurveda uses Ashwagandha (Withania somnifera) and Brahmi (Bacopa monnieri) for their potential stress-reducing and brain-enhancing benefits. Yoga and meditation can help manage cravings and reduce anxiety.

The integration of modern medicine, Ayurveda, and yoga can offer a multifaceted approach to treatment. This holistic strategy leverages the strengths of each discipline, potentially enhancing overall patient wellbeing. However, it's essential to consult with healthcare professionals before starting or modifying any treatment plan.

IMPACT of INTEGRATION

The integration of modern medicine, yoga, and Ayurveda offers an enriched, holistic approach to health care that could greatly benefit individuals, families, communities, and the entire nation. A comprehensive care model incorporating these practices can provide a more well-rounded approach to health and wellness.

For patients, this integrated approach can lead to improved health outcomes. Modern medicine, with its evidence-based practice, excels in the treatment of acute conditions and surgical interventions. By integrating yoga and Ayurveda, patients can also tap into holistic methods that emphasize the prevention of disease and the maintenance of health, leading to overall well-being. Yoga, in particular, is a mind-body practice that can reduce stress, improve mental health, enhance physical fitness, and increase body awareness. When integrated into a health care regimen, yoga can help manage chronic conditions, reduce the side effects of treatment, and improve the quality of life for patients. Ayurveda, a traditional Indian system of medicine, aims at maintaining health through balancing the body's energies. The system provides natural remedies and lifestyle modifications that can complement modern medical treatment. For example, the dietary advice and herbal medicines of Ayurveda can provide support to the digestive system and strengthen the body's natural defences.

For families, the integration of these practices can mean a healthier household. Yoga and Ayurvedic practices can be easily incorporated into daily routines, promoting health and preventing disease for all family members. Additionally, Ayurveda's emphasis on diet and nutrition can lead to healthier eating habits for the entire family.

From a societal perspective, promoting health and preventing disease can lead to a healthier community overall. It's well known that healthy individuals contribute to healthier communities. As yoga and Ayurveda emphasize the promotion of health, they can help create communities with lower disease burdens. A healthier community means fewer hospital visits, less burden on health care facilities, and lower health care costs. This is particularly significant in managing chronic diseases, which are a major driver of health care costs. The holistic and preventative focus of yoga and Ayurveda can play a key role in controlling these long-term conditions.

This integrated approach also holds the potential for increased productivity in the workplace. Healthy employees are less likely to take sick leaves, are more productive, and contribute positively to the overall performance of the organization. This is beneficial for both the employer and the employee. The practice of yoga and Ayurveda, which includes meditation and relaxation techniques, can help reduce stress and improve mental well-being. This is particularly significant in today's fast-paced society where stress-related disorders are prevalent. Improved mental health can result in more positive social interactions, fostering stronger communities.

The integration of modern medicine, yoga, and Ayurveda can also enhance health literacy and empower individuals to take charge of their health. By learning about these practices, individuals can make informed decisions about their health and adopt practices that foster well-being. With health being a key contributor to the quality of life, this integrated approach can improve living standards. Better health means more active participation in social activities, fostering a more vibrant community life.

At the national level, reducing the disease burden can translate to significant cost savings. Health care expenditure is a major concern for any country. By preventing diseases and promoting health, we can reduce the need for expensive treatments and hospitalizations. Healthier individuals also mean a healthier workforce. This can lead to increased productivity, positively impacting the country's economic growth. This is particularly significant for countries with a large working-age population.

The growth of yoga and Ayurveda can lead to increased demand for trained professionals in these fields. This can contribute to job creation and economic growth. The integration of modern medicine, yoga, and Ayurveda also holds potential for tourism. Health and wellness tourism is a growing industry globally. By promoting these practices, countries can attract health-conscious tourists. This integrated approach can also foster cultural preservation. Yoga and Ayurveda are ancient practices with rich cultural heritage. Their integration into mainstream health care can help preserve and promote these traditions.

At the global level, the integration of modern medicine, yoga, and Ayurveda can contribute to the achievement of the Sustainable Development Goals, particularly the goal of ensuring healthy lives and promoting well-being for all.

To realize these benefits, it's important to address the challenges involved in integrating these systems. This includes the need for rigorous scientific research to validate the efficacy and safety of yoga and Ayurvedic practices, standardization of these practices, and training of professionals. It's also necessary to increase awareness about these practices. Public health campaigns, incorporating yoga and Ayurveda into school curricula, and promoting these practices in workplaces can be effective strategies.

In this way, the integration of modern medicine, yoga, and Ayurveda can lead to improved health outcomes, promote health and prevent disease, reduce health care costs, and contribute to economic growth. This requires collective efforts from individuals, health professionals, communities, and policymakers. With commitment and collaboration, we can harness the strengths of these systems for better health and well-being.

COST-BENEFIT ANALYSIS

Integrating modern medicine, yoga, and Ayurveda may have significant cost-saving implications. For one, Ayurveda and yoga focus on prevention and maintenance of health, which could result in fewer incidences of serious illness and therefore reduce the need for expensive treatments and hospitalizations.

Real Costs: According to a report published by the American Journal of Health Promotion, yoga practice was linked to approximately $3,000 in annual savings per person on medical services. The preventative nature of yoga could help avert chronic diseases that are costly to treat and manage.

Estimating Healthcare Cost Savings in the UK is slightly difficult because the National Health Service (NHS) in the UK is publicly funded. The increasing burden of chronic diseases like diabetes, cardiovascular diseases, mental health disorders is continually escalating the NHS expenditure. By incorporating preventive and holistic approaches like Yoga and Ayurveda, it could help decrease the incidence of such chronic diseases, resulting in significant cost savings for the NHS. The integration of Yoga and Ayurveda with modern medicine will lead to significant Improvement in Mental Health. In the UK, mental health problems represent the largest single cause of disability, with the cost of mental ill health estimated at £105 billion a year. Yoga is shown to have considerable benefits for mental health, including reduction of stress, anxiety, and depression. Incorporating regular yoga practices could potentially lead to savings in mental health treatments. Mental health problems are also a significant cause of economic loss due to decreased productivity. By helping to improve mental health, yoga can contribute to increased workplace productivity and decreased health care costs. Some of the examples for cost saving are given below:

Diabetes

Diabetes care represents a significant cost for the NHS, estimated at £10 billion per year. Yoga has shown promising results in controlling blood sugar levels and improving insulin sensitivity. In Ayurveda, plants like Gymnema sylvestre and Pterocarpus marsupium have been used for thousands of years to help control blood sugar. Implementing yoga and Ayurveda as complementary therapies could help control diabetes progression and complications, potentially reducing the cost associated with long-term care.

Hypertension

The NHS spends an estimated £2 billion per year on hypertension-related health costs. Yoga is known for its positive effects on reducing stress and blood pressure. Ayurveda also uses various herbs like Rauwolfia serpentina, known for their blood pressure-lowering effects. Integrating these practices into a comprehensive treatment plan could aid in reducing the overall costs associated with managing hypertension.

Anxiety Disorders

Anxiety disorders, including panic disorder and generalized anxiety disorder, are estimated to cost the NHS about £1.2 billion annually. Both yoga and Ayurveda can offer significant relief from symptoms of anxiety. Yoga promotes relaxation and stress reduction, while Ayurvedic treatments focus on balancing the body's energies (doshas) using diet, lifestyle, and herbal remedies like Ashwagandha. Together, they may be able to decrease reliance on costly pharmacological treatments.

Depression

The economic burden of depression on the NHS is enormous, estimated at £2.4 billion annually. Yoga has been found to enhance mood and act as an effective adjunct treatment for depression. Similarly, Ayurveda uses natural remedies, such as the herb St John's Wort, to help balance mood and alleviate depressive symptoms. With the integration of these treatments, it may be possible to reduce the overall expenditure on managing depression.

Dementia and Alzheimer's Disease

Dementia and Alzheimer's disease are estimated to cost the NHS approximately £5 billion per year. Evidence suggests that yoga can enhance cognitive function and reduce stress, which can help delay the onset of dementia. Ayurvedic medicine, using herbs like Turmeric and Brahmi, may also help improve cognitive function. Incorporating these therapies could help reduce the economic burden of these diseases.

This synopsis shows that the integration of yoga and Ayurveda with conventional treatments can potentially alleviate the economic burden on the NHS. However, more in-depth research and larger clinical trials are needed to conclusively prove the benefits and cost-effectiveness of these approaches.

Chronic Fatigue Syndrome

Chronic Fatigue Syndrome (CFS), also known as myalgic encephalomyelitis (ME), is estimated to cost the NHS around £3.3 billion annually. CFS is a complex disorder, and management is largely supportive, involving a combination of medications, cognitive behavioural therapy (CBT), and graded exercise therapy (GET). Yoga's focus on gentle movement and mindfulness can complement these therapies, helping to manage symptoms and improve quality of life. Certain Ayurvedic practices and herbs, like Ashwagandha and Brahmi, are also known for their adaptogenic and nerve-tonic properties, potentially beneficial for CFS patients.

Fibromyalgia

Fibromyalgia's annual cost to the NHS is estimated at £3.8 billion. This chronic pain disorder is often challenging to manage with conventional medicine alone. Yoga's gentle stretching, deep breathing, and mindfulness may help manage pain and fatigue associated with fibromyalgia. Additionally, Ayurvedic treatments focused on balancing the doshas and managing stress, along with herbs like Boswellia, could provide added benefits.

Attention Deficit Hyperactivity Disorder (ADHD)

The estimated annual cost of ADHD to the NHS is approximately £900 million. While stimulant medication is a first-line treatment, yoga and Ayurveda could provide adjunctive support. Yoga's focus on breath control, meditation, and physical postures can help improve concentration, while Ayurvedic treatments such as dietary changes, lifestyle recommendations, and herbs like Brahmi may help balance energies, leading to improved focus and behavior.

Osteoarthritis

Osteoarthritis costs the NHS about £5.2 billion annually. Yoga's gentle, weight-bearing exercises can help improve joint health and mobility. Ayurvedic treatments, such as topical and oral use of herbs like Turmeric and Ashwagandha, can provide pain relief and reduce inflammation, potentially reducing the need for expensive surgeries.

Osteoporosis

The annual cost of treating osteoporosis and related fractures to the NHS is around £4.5 billion. Weight-bearing exercises, including certain yoga postures, can help improve bone density. Ayurvedic treatments may include calcium-rich herbal supplements, dietary changes, and lifestyle recommendations, potentially delaying the progression of the disease and reducing the risk of fractures.

Chronic Pain

Chronic pain is another major health issue, costing the NHS an estimated £10 billion each year. Chronic pain conditions can often be difficult to treat effectively with conventional medicine alone, leading to high direct medical costs and indirect costs such as lost productivity. Yoga has been found to be beneficial in managing various types of chronic pain, including lower back pain, neck pain, and fibromyalgia. Additionally, Ayurvedic therapies can provide a complementary approach to pain management, potentially reducing the need for high-cost interventions such as surgery or long-term use of opioid painkillers.

Looking at just these few disease conditions it can be said that the integration of yoga and Ayurveda with conventional modern medicine can offer significant potential cost savings for the health services in managing chronic diseases. This approach could reduce reliance on high-cost treatments, minimize side effects, improve patient quality of life, and result in better overall health outcomes

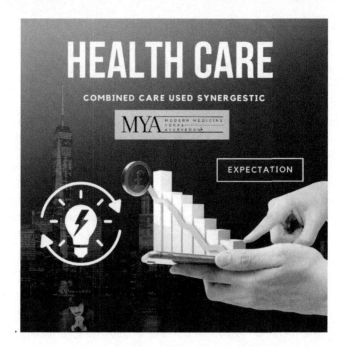

However, further research is needed to fully quantify the cost benefits and to determine the best methods for implementing these practices into mainstream healthcare in the Uk and other countries.

> Integrating yoga and Ayurveda with conventional medical treatment for these chronic diseases could potentially lead to cost savings for the NHS. However, more research is needed to determine the full extent of potential savings and to develop best practices for integrative care.

Indirect Cost Benefits:

Productivity Gains: According to a study published in the Journal of Occupational Health, work-related stress, depression, or anxiety accounted for 51% of all work-related ill health cases and 55% of all working days lost due to work-related ill health in the UK in 2019/20. As Yoga and Ayurveda help in stress management and overall well-being, they can contribute to reduced work absenteeism and increased productivity, leading to economic benefits.

Prevention of Lifestyle Diseases: Lifestyle diseases like diabetes, obesity, and cardiovascular diseases are on the rise in the UK. Yoga and Ayurveda's emphasis on a balanced lifestyle and diet could potentially reduce the incidence of such diseases, leading to considerable cost savings in healthcare and improved quality of life.

Ayurveda also facilitates lifestyle and dietary changes, the impact of which on overall health cannot be underestimated. Many chronic illnesses such as diabetes, heart disease, and certain types of cancer are linked to lifestyle and dietary choices. By implementing changes suggested by Ayurveda, it's possible to decrease the prevalence of these diseases, thereby leading to significant cost savings.

Quality of Life: Although challenging to quantify in monetary terms, the improved quality of life brought about by regular yoga practice and adherence to Ayurveda principles—such as increased energy, better mood, improved sleep quality—can lead to less quantifiable but arguably equally valuable societal benefits. The benefits include factors such as increased energy, better mood, improved sleep quality, and general well-being, which are often reported with the regular practice of yoga and adherence to Ayurvedic principles.

Costs of Integration: Costs of integration would include training healthcare providers in Yoga and Ayurveda, public education, and potentially more time spent per patient in the healthcare system. These should be compared against the potential cost savings from prevention of diseases, decreased need for expensive treatments, and increased productivity.

Full cost-effectiveness of integrating modern medicine, yoga, and Ayurveda is complex and should be examined through rigorous, comprehensive economic evaluation. This includes considering all costs and benefits, both direct and indirect, and conducting long-term follow-up to understand the sustained impact of this approach on health and health care costs.

While the direct costs of implementing such integrative programs may be clear, quantifying the indirect cost savings can be challenging. More research is needed to understand the long-term economic impact of this integrative approach. This research should consider not just the cost of healthcare services, but also the impact on productivity, quality of life, and societal wellbeing.

We can thus see that the integration of modern medicine, yoga, and Ayurveda has the potential to provide cost-effective solutions for the prevention and management of disease. By promoting health and preventing disease, we can reduce the demand for expensive treatments, thereby lowering the overall cost of healthcare. However, more research is needed to fully understand the economic implications of this integrative approach.

References:

1. Curtis, L., & Burns, A. (2018). Unit Costs of Health and Social Care 2018. Canterbury: Personal Social Services Research Unit, University of Kent. This report is produced annually and provides details about the unit costs of a wide range of health and social care services in the UK.
2. Department of Health and Social Care. (2013). Reference costs 2012 to 2013. Available at: https://www.gov.uk/government/publications/nhs-reference-costs-2012-to-2013 This document provides detailed information on the costs of different NHS services.
3. National Institute for Health and Care Excellence. (2013). Guide to the methods of technology appraisal 2013. London: NICE. This guide outlines the methods used by NICE to undertake cost-effectiveness analyses of health technologies.

4. Larg, A., & Moss, J. R. (2011). Cost-of-illness studies: a guide to critical evaluation. Pharmacoeconomics, 29(8), 653-671. This article provides a guide for the critical evaluation of cost-of-illness studies.

5. Department of Health. (2011). NHS reference costs 2010 to 2011. Available at: https://www.gov.uk/government/publications/nhs-reference-costs-2010-to-2011 Another source of detailed information on the costs of different NHS services.

6. Drummond, M. F., Sculpher, M. J., Claxton, K., Stoddart, G. L., & Torrance, G. W. (2015). Methods for the economic evaluation of health care programmes. Oxford university press. This is a comprehensive textbook on the methods and techniques used in economic evaluation in health care.

7. Office for National Statistics (ONS). Health accounts: UK Health Accounts: 2017. Available at: https://www.ons.gov.uk/releases/ukhealthaccounts2017 This data gives an insight into UK healthcare expenditure, including diseases and conditions, and is compiled to international definitions set out in the System of Health Accounts 2011.

8. Barnett K, Mercer SW, Norbury M, Watt G, Wyke S, Guthrie B. (2012). Epidemiology of multimorbidity and implications for health care, research, and medical education: a cross-sectional study. Lancet. 380(9836):37-43.

9. Briggs, A., Claxton, K., & Sculpher, M. (2006). Decision Modelling for Health Economic Evaluation. Oxford University Press. A comprehensive guide to decision modelling, a critical component of health economic evaluations.

10. National Health Service (NHS). (2020). Annual Report and Accounts 2019/20. Available at: https://www.england.nhs.uk/publication/nhs-england-annual-report-and-accounts-2019-20/ This report provides information about NHS England's performance and financial position for the year 2019/20.

11. National Institute for Health and Care Excellence (NICE). (2020). Costing statement: Implementing NICE guidance. Available at: https://www.nice.org.uk/guidance/ph38/resources/costing-statement-pdf-69120453 This NICE statement provides estimates of the national cost impact arising from implementing guidance.

12. Hancock, R., King, J., & Maloney, J. (2020). The cost of poor mental health to UK employers. Centre for Mental Health. This report provides insight into the impact and cost of poor mental health on UK employers, which can inform broader understandings of cost in the healthcare context.

13. Office for National Statistics (ONS). (2020). Health state life expectancies by national deprivation deciles, England and Wales: 2017 to 2019. Available at: https://www.ons.gov.uk/peoplepopulationandcommunity/healthandsocialcare/healthandlifeexpectancies/bulletins/healthstatelifeexpectanciesbynationaldeprivationdecilesenglandandwales/2017to2019 This report provides statistics on health state life expectancies by deprivation deciles, offering insight into health disparities and their potential cost implications.

14. Public Health England. (2021). Health matters: Health economics – making the most of your budget. Available at: https://www.gov.uk/government/publications/health-matters-health-economics-making-the-most-of-your-budget/health-matters-health-economics-making-the-most-of-your-budget This resource provides information on health economics and guides how to make the most of a healthcare budget.

15. Iacobucci, G. (2019). NHS is urged to publish the cost of its drugs. BMJ, 364, l196. This paper highlights the need for transparency in the costs of drugs used by the NHS.

16. McCrone, P., Dhanasiri, S., Patel, A., Knapp, M., & Lawton-Smith, S. (2008). Paying the Price: The cost of mental health care in England to 2026. King's Fund. This report projects the costs of mental health care in England up to 2026, providing important data on potential future expenditure.

17. Hex, N., Bartlett, C., Wright, D., Taylor, M., & Varley, D. (2012). Estimating the current and future costs of Type 1 and Type 2 diabetes in the UK, including direct health costs and indirect societal and productivity costs. Diabetic Medicine, 29(7), 855-862. A study that estimates the current and future costs of Type 1 and Type 2 diabetes in the UK.

18. ONS. (2020). Costs of healthcare for the adult population: 2015 to 2017. Available at: https://www.ons.gov.uk/peoplepopulationandcommunity/healthandsocialcare/healthcare system/articles/costsofhealthcarefortheadultpopulation/2015to2017 This article presents the estimated costs of healthcare for the adult population by age and sex, providing detailed data to help understand expenditure distribution.

19. Curtis, L., & Burns, A. (2020). Unit Costs of Health and Social Care 2020. Personal Social Services Research Unit, University of Kent, Canterbury. This report provides up-to-date information about the costs of health and social care in the UK.

20. Bevan, G., Karanikolos, M., Exley, J., Nolte, E., Connolly, S., & Mays, N. (2014). The four health systems of the United Kingdom: How do they compare? Nuffield Trust. A comprehensive comparison of the four health systems of the United Kingdom, which provides insights into the varying costs and outcomes across the different systems.

21. Davies, S. C. (2014). Annual Report of the Chief Medical Officer 2013, Public Mental Health Priorities: Investing in the Evidence. Department of Health. This report highlights the key public mental health priorities and the associated costs, emphasising the importance of investing in evidence-based approaches.

22. Raftery, J. (2001). NICE: faster access to modern t eatments? Analysis of guidance on health technologies. BMJ, 323(7324), 1300-1303. A report on how the National Institute for Health and Clinical Excellence (NICE) has impacted the accessibility and cost-effectiveness of health technologies in the UK.

23. Barbieri, M., Drummond, M., Rutten, F., Cook, J., Glick, H., Lis, J., Reed, S. D., & Sculpher, M. (2010). What do international pharmacoeconomic guidelines say about economic data transferability? Value in Health, 13(8), 1028-1037. An examination of international pharmacoeconomic guidelines on the transferability of economic data, a key factor when considering cost analyses across different countries or healthcare systems.

24. National Institute for Health and Care Excellence (NICE). (2013). Guide to the methods of technology appraisal 2013. Available at: https://www.nice.org.uk/process/pmg9/resources/guide-to-the-methods-of-technology-appraisal-2013-pdf-2007975843781 This guide outlines the methods of technology appraisal used by NICE, which plays a crucial role in determining cost-effectiveness and affordability in the UK healthcare system.

25. Briggs, A. H., Weinstein, M. C., Fenwick, E. A., Karnon, J., Sculpher, M. J., & Paltiel, A. D. (2012). Model parameter estimation and uncertainty analysis: a report of the ISPOR-SMDM Modeling Good Research Practices Task Force Working Group–6. Medical decision making, 32(5), 722-732. A report that discusses model parameter estimation and uncertainty analysis, two key aspects of understanding and interpreting cost data in healthcare.

SUMMARY

The strength of modern medicine is well-established, with its precise diagnostic tools, powerful drugs, and sophisticated surgeries. However, it's increasingly recognized that this approach can sometimes be reductionist, focusing on specific diseases and symptoms without always considering the broader context of an individual's health and lifestyle. That's where yoga and Ayurveda, ancient systems of well-being, come in. When combined, these three offer an integrative, holistic approach to health that can not only treat diseases but also promote wellness and prevent future health issues.

Cardiovascular health is a global concern with heart disease being a leading cause of death. Modern medicine offers various interventions like statins for cholesterol management, antihypertensives, and surgeries. However, these don't address underlying lifestyle factors that often drive these diseases. Yoga, with its emphasis on physical activity and stress reduction, has been shown to improve cardiovascular health. Ayurveda, through dietary recommendations and natural remedies, also supports heart health. Combining these with modern treatments can provide a more comprehensive approach to cardiovascular care.

Respiratory disorders like asthma and COPD can significantly affect a person's quality of life. While modern medicine provides drugs to manage symptoms, yoga offers breathing techniques that improve lung capacity and function. Ayurveda can help identify and mitigate dietary and environmental triggers of respiratory issues. Together, these three approaches can help patients manage symptoms more effectively.

Neurological disorders such as Parkinson's, Alzheimer's, and multiple sclerosis pose significant challenges for modern medicine due to their complex nature. Yoga's focus on mindfulness and physical stability can enhance mental health and mobility, while Ayurvedic practices can support overall neurological health. When combined with conventional treatments, these can enhance quality of life for those with neurological conditions.

Digestive disorders can be deeply affected by diet and lifestyle, areas often addressed inadequately by modern medicine. Ayurveda, with its emphasis on healthy dietary practices, can provide natural remedies and personalized diet plans, while yoga can improve digestion through physical postures. This integrative approach can offer a more holistic treatment for digestive disorders.

Endocrine disorders like diabetes and thyroid disorders are rising globally. Modern medicine offers hormone replacement therapy and other treatments, but these often have side effects. Yoga, through its stress-reducing and hormone-regulating effects, can support endocrine health. Ayurveda provides dietary and herbal solutions for these disorders. Integrating these with modern medicine can result in more comprehensive and effective care.

For reproductive health, the combination of modern medicine, yoga, and Ayurveda is promising. While modern medicine provides hormonal treatments and surgeries, yoga can enhance fertility and sexual health through specific postures and stress reduction. Ayurveda's emphasis on diet and lifestyle can improve reproductive health and fertility. This integrated approach can provide a well-rounded treatment strategy for both male and female reproductive issues.

Skin disorders like eczema, psoriasis, and acne often require long-term management. Modern medicine offers topical and systemic treatments, but these can have side effects. Yoga's stress-reducing effects can benefit skin health, and Ayurveda offers dietary advice and natural remedies. An integrated approach can provide a more holistic and sustainable solution for skin disorders.

Haematological conditions like anaemia and clotting disorders can be life-altering. Modern medicine provides blood transfusions and drugs, but these can have side effects and don't always address underlying issues. Yoga can improve circulation, and Ayurveda can offer dietary advice to support blood health. An integrative approach can offer a broader solution for these disorders.

Infectious diseases and immune disorders pose a significant challenge for modern medicine. While antibiotics and other drugs are critical, they don't support the immune system. Yoga's stress-reducing and immune-enhancing benefits can support immune health, and Ayurveda offers dietary and herbal interventions to enhance immunity. Combining these with modern treatments can offer a more comprehensive approach to infectious and immune conditions.

Lastly, reproductive problems like infertility, menstrual disorders, and menopausal symptoms can be complex. Modern medicine offers hormonal therapies and assisted reproductive technologies, but these can be invasive and have side effects. Yoga can support reproductive health through stress reduction and hormone balance, and Ayurveda offers dietary and lifestyle interventions. An integrated approach can provide a more personalized and holistic treatment for these problems.

The combination of modern medicine, yoga, and Ayurveda for disease treatment and prevention offers a patient-centered, comprehensive approach. It combines the best of scientific advances with ancient wisdom, addressing not just the disease but the whole person. It has the potential to improve health outcomes, patient satisfaction, and overall health care.

However, this integration requires an open mind, respect for different health philosophies, and the willingness to learn from each other. It involves patients, doctors, and health systems embracing a more holistic vision of health. It calls for research to understand how these approaches can best complement each other, and for regulatory systems that support this integration.

Importantly, this integrative approach does not mean abandoning modern medicine. Rather, it means expanding our health toolbox, combining the best of different health traditions. It means recognizing that health is more than the absence of disease and that lifestyle plays a crucial role in our well-being.

Ultimately, the integration of modern medicine, yoga, and Ayurveda has the potential to create a more comprehensive, holistic, and patient-centered approach to health care. By treating the individual rather than just the disease, it can improve health outcomes, enhance patient satisfaction, and potentially reduce health care costs.

References List

Here is the list of important additional references used to compile this book. They are a great resource if you wish to explore the topics discussed in more detail.

1. Mayo Clinic Staff. (2021). Modern vs. Alternative Medicine: What's the difference? Mayo Clinic.
2. Feuerstein, G. (2012). The Yoga Tradition: Its History, Literature, Philosophy, and Practice. Hohm Press.
3. Lad, V. (2002). Textbook of Ayurveda: Fundamental Principles. Ayurvedic Press.
4. Tirtha, S. S. (1998). The Ayurveda Encyclopedia: Natural Secrets to Healing, Prevention & Longevity. Ayurveda Holistic Center Press.
5. Khalsa, S.B.S., Cohen, L., McCall, T., & Telles, S. (2016). The Principles and Practice of Yoga in Health Care. Handspring Publishing.
6. McCall, T. (2007). Yoga as Medicine: The Yogic Prescription for Health and Healing. Bantam.
7. National Center for Complementary and Integrative Health (2021). Yoga: What You Need to Know. U.S. Department of Health & Human Services.
8. Johns Hopkins Medicine. (2021). The Science of Yoga. Johns Hopkins Medicine.
9. Pizzorno, J. E., Murray, M. T., & Joiner-Bey, H. (2016). The Clinician's Handbook of Natural Medicine. Churchill Livingstone.
10. Selby, A. (2021). Yoga and Ayurveda: Self-Healing and Self-Realization. Lotus Press.
11. Mishra, L.C. (2003). Scientific Basis for Ayurvedic Therapies. CRC Press.
12. Dass, V. (1999). Ayurvedic Health Practitioner Textbook. Vasant Lad.
13. Birdee, G.S., Legedza, A.T., Saper, R.B., Bertisch, S.M., Eisenberg, D.M., & Phillips, R.S. (2008). Characteristics of Yoga Users: Results of a National Survey. Journal of General Internal Medicine, 23(10), 1653–1658.
14. Balasubramaniam, M., Telles, S., & Doraiswamy, P. M. (2013). Yoga on Our Minds: A Systematic Review of Yoga for Neuropsychiatric Disorders. Frontiers in Psychiatry, 3, 117.
15. Telles, S., Singh, N., & Balkrishna, A. (2012). Managing Mental Health Disorders Resulting from Trauma through Yoga: A Review. Depression Research and Treatment, 2012, 401513.
16. Ward, L., Stebbings, S., Cherkin, D., & Baxter, G.D. (2013). Yoga for Functional Ability, Pain and Psychosocial Outcomes in Musculoskeletal Conditions: A Systematic Review and Meta-Analysis. Musculoskeletal Care, 11(4), 203–217.
17. Rastogi, S., & Kaphle, K. (2010). Complementary and Alternative Medicine in Cancer Pain Management: A Systematic Review. Indian Journal of Palliative Care, 16(1), 1–15.

18. National Center for Complementary and Integrative Health (2020). Ayurvedic Medicine: In Depth. U.S. Department of Health & Human Services.
19. Patwardhan, B. (2014). Bridging Ayurveda with Evidence-Based Scientific Approaches in Medicine. The EPMA Journal, 5(1), 19.
20. Chatterjee, B., & Pancholi, J. (2011). Pragmatic and Personalized Approach to Treatment of Disease: The Role of Ayurveda. Personalized Medicine, 8(1), 67–75.
21. The Chopra Center. (2021). What is Ayurveda? The Chopra Center.
22. Mayo Clinic Staff. (2021). Integrative Medicine: Find Out What Works. Mayo Clinic.
23. Coulter, I.D., & Willis, E.M. (2004). The Rise and Rise of Complementary and Alternative Medicine: A Sociological Perspective. Medical Journal of Australia, 180(11), 587–589.
24. Bell, I.R., Caspi, O., Schwartz, G.E., Grant, K.L., Gaudet, T.W., Rychener, D., Maizes, V., & Weil, A. (2002). Integrative Medicine and Systemic Outcomes Research: Issues in the Emergence of a New Model for Primary Health Care. Archives of Internal Medicine, 162(2), 133–140.
25. Mehta, P., & Dhapte, V. (2015). Milestones in the History of Yoga and Ayurveda in the Twentieth Century. International Journal of Yoga, 8(2), 160–163.
26. Maizes, V., Rakel, D., & Niemiec, C. (2009). Integrative Medicine and Patient-Centered Care. Explore (New York, N.Y.), 5(5), 277–289.
27. Tricot, O., Tricot, S., Leheup, B., Georger, F., Boyaval, M., & François, M. (2020). Lifestyle and Dietary Factors in Relation to Cardiovascular Health: a Citizens' Jury. Patient Preference and Adherence, 14, 119–128.
28. Stussman, B., Black, L., Barnes, P., Clarke, T., & Nahin, R. (2015). Wellness-related Use of Common Complementary Health Approaches Among Adults: United States, 2012. National Health Statistics Reports, (85), 1–12.
29. Wieland, L.S., Manheimer, E., & Berman, B.M. (2011). Development and Classification of an Operational Definition of Complementary and Alternative Medicine for the Cochrane Collaboration. Alternative Therapies in Health and Medicine, 17(2), 50–59.
30. Templeman, K., Robinson, A., & McKenna, L. (2015). A Systematic Review of the Physical Health Impacts from Non-Occupational Exposure to Wildfire Smoke. Environmental Research, 136, 120–132.

Glossary

Modern Medicine: Also known as Western medicine or Allopathy, it is a system of health care that aims to prevent, diagnose, and treat diseases through scientifically tested and proven methods such as medications, surgery, and other treatments.

Yoga: Originating from ancient India, yoga is a holistic practice encompassing physical postures, breathing exercises, meditation, and ethical principles. It aims to promote physical health, mental clarity, emotional balance, and spiritual growth.

Ayurveda: An ancient system of medicine from India, Ayurveda emphasizes disease prevention and health promotion through a balanced lifestyle, dietary practices, herbal remedies, body therapies, and mental and spiritual nurturing. The term is derived from the Sanskrit words 'Ayur' (life) and 'Veda' (science or knowledge), meaning 'the science of life'.

Integrative medicine approach: This approach to healthcare incorporates the best of different health modalities (including modern medicine, yoga, and Ayurveda) to provide personalized, holistic care. It addresses the full range of physical, emotional, mental, social, spiritual, and environmental influences that affect health.

Holistic: A perspective that views the body, mind, and spirit as interconnected and integral aspects of a person's overall health and wellbeing.

Dosha: In Ayurveda, doshas are the three energies (Vata, Pitta, and Kapha) that govern physiological activity in the body, each with its specific physical and psychological characteristics. These are believed to circulate in the body and govern physiological activity.

Patient-centred Care: A healthcare approach that respects and responds to individual patient preferences, needs, and values, ensuring that patient values guide all clinical decisions.

Personalized Medicine: An approach that tailors medical treatment to the individual characteristics of each patient.

MYA – Modern Medicine, Yoga and Ayurveda combined approach

Vata: One of the three doshas, associated with movement, thought, and communication. It's composed of the elements air and space.

Pitta: One of the three doshas, associated with metabolism, digestion, and transformation. It's composed of the elements fire and water.

Kapha: One of the three doshas, associated with structure, stability, and lubrication. It's composed of the elements earth and water.

Prakriti: An individual's unique constitution or "nature," determined by the balance of the three doshas at the time of conception.

Agni: The metabolic fire that governs digestion and metabolism in the body.

Ama: Toxins produced in the body due to improper digestion.

Ojas: The essence of all bodily tissues, responsible for overall strength, immunity, and vitality.

Sattva: One of the three gunas or qualities, sattva is associated with purity, knowledge, and harmony.

Rajas: One of the three gunas, rajas is associated with action, passion, and movement.

Tamas: One of the three gunas, tamas is associated with inertia, darkness, and ignorance.

Dhatus: The seven fundamental tissues of the body: plasma, blood, muscle, fat, bone, marrow/nerve, and reproductive tissue.

Prana: The life force or vital energy that flows in the body.

Chakras: The seven major energy centers aligned along the spine, starting at the base and ending at the crown of the head.

Nadis: The channels through which the energies of the subtle body flow. The three primary nadis are the Ida, Pingala, and Sushumna.

Ida: The nadi associated with the left side of the body, moon energy, and cooling, calming actions.

Pingala: The nadi associated with the right side of the body, sun energy, and warming, stimulating actions.

Sushumna: The central nadi that runs along the spinal column, where kundalini energy is said to rise.

Kundalini: A form of primal energy said to be located at the base of the spine.

Dinacharya: The daily routine recommended by Ayurveda to align with the natural rhythms of the day.

Ritucharya: The seasonal routine recommended by Ayurveda to align with the changing energies of nature throughout the year.

Abhyanga: A form of Ayurvedic therapy that involves massage with large amounts of warm oil.

Marma Points: The vital points in the body where the subtle prana energy is transformed, distributed, or redirected.

Panchakarma: A set of five therapeutic treatments used in Ayurvedic medicine for cleansing the body of toxins.

Virechana: A part of the Panchakarma procedure that involves purgation or elimination therapy to remove toxins from the body.

Basti: An Ayurvedic therapy that involves the introduction of herbal decoctions in a liquid medium into the rectum to cleanse the body of toxins.

Nasya: An Ayurvedic therapy that involves the application of medicated oils to the nostrils to cleanse the head and neck of toxins.

Rasayana: Ayurvedic rejuvenation therapy aimed at promoting vitality and longevity.

Shirodhara: A form of Ayurvedic therapy that involves gently pouring liquids, usually oil, over the forehead.

Netra Tarpana: An Ayurvedic therapy for the eyes, it involves bathing the eyes in ghee.

Triphala: A traditional Ayurvedic formulation made from three fruits: Amalaki, Bibhitaki, and Haritaki.

Amalaki (Emblica officinalis): A fruit used in Ayurveda known for its rejuvenating properties and high Vitamin C content.

Haritaki (Terminalia chebula): A fruit used in Ayurveda known for its rejuvenating properties and ability to support healthy bowel movement.

Bibhitaki (Terminalia bellirica): A fruit used in Ayurveda known for its rejuvenating properties and ability to support respiratory health.

Ashwagandha (Withania somnifera): A root used in Ayurveda as an adaptogen to help the body cope with stress.

Brahmi (Bacopa monnieri): A herb used in Ayurveda to improve brain functions like memory, concentration, and cognition.

Tulsi (Ocimum sanctum): A herb used in Ayurveda for its adaptogenic and immune-supportive properties.

Turmeric (Curcuma longa): A root used in Ayurveda for its anti-inflammatory and antioxidant properties.

Ghee: Clarified butter, used in Ayurveda as a cooking medium and a substance in various therapies.

Kitchari: A traditional Ayurvedic dish made from mung beans and rice, used for its easy digestibility and detoxifying properties.

Chyawanprash: An Ayurvedic herbal jam packed with a multitude of herbs, used as a tonic for overall health and vitality.

Shatavari (Asparagus racemosus): A plant used in Ayurveda known for its rejuvenative properties, particularly for the female reproductive system.

Arjuna (Terminalia arjuna): A tree bark used in Ayurveda known for its cardiovascular benefits.

Neem (Azadirachta indica): A plant used in Ayurveda for its purifying and detoxifying properties.

Tagara (Valeriana wallichii): A root used in Ayurveda for its calming and sleep-promoting properties.

Bhumyamalaki (Phyllanthus niruri): A plant used in Ayurveda for its liver-supportive properties.

Manjistha (Rubia cordifolia): A plant used in Ayurveda for its blood-purifying properties.

Guduchi (Tinospora cordifolia): A herb used in Ayurveda for its immune-supportive properties.

Shilajit: A resin used in Ayurveda known for its rejuvenating and revitalizing properties.

Pranayama: Breathing exercises designed to control the prana or life force.

Surya Namaskar: A sequence of 12 powerful yoga poses with profound benefits that enhance the overall posture and flexibility of the body.

Atman: The individual soul or self, often used in the context of one's true self beyond the ego.

Bhakti: Devotion or love for a higher power, often expressed through practices such as chanting, prayer, and rituals.

Jnana: Knowledge or wisdom, often used in the context of spiritual knowledge or enlightenment.

Karma: The law of cause and effect, the belief that every action has an equal reaction.

Dharma: Duty or virtue, the moral and ethical duties that need to be followed for a harmonious life.

Moksha: Liberation or release, often used in the context of spiritual liberation from the cycle of birth and death.

Ahimsa: Non-violence or non-harm, a central tenet of Ayurveda and yoga, extended to thoughts, words, and actions.

Satya: Truthfulness, another core tenet of Ayurveda and yoga.

Brahmacharya: The practice of celibacy or right use of energy, often associated with control of sensual pleasures.

Aparigraha: Non-greed or non-attachment, the practice of contentment and letting go.

Svadhyaya: Self-study or self-reflection, a practice of introspection and self-understanding.

Asana: The physical postures practiced in yoga.

Dhyana: Meditation, a practice of focusing the mind to achieve mental clarity and emotional calmness.

Samadhi: The ultimate state of concentration or superconsciousness achieved through meditation.

Samskara: Mental and emotional patterns or imprints that influence our actions and experiences.

Niyama: The second limb of yoga, referring to personal observances towards oneself.

Yama: The first limb of yoga, referring to ethical standards or moral disciplines.

Rasa: The taste or essence of food, also used to describe the various stages of digestion in the body.

Vipaka: The post-digestive effect of food or herbs on the body.

Virya: The potency or energy of food or herbs.

Churna: Powdered herbs or spices used in Ayurvedic medicine.

Vati: Tablets or pills in Ayurvedic medicine, made from herbal powders or extracts.

Avaleha: Herbal jams or pastes used in Ayurvedic medicine.

Ghruta: Medicated ghee, used as a vehicle for delivering the medicinal properties of herbs.

Kashaya: Herbal decoctions used in Ayurvedic medicine.

Lepa: Herbal pastes applied externally for therapeutic purposes.

Agni Karma: An Ayurvedic treatment involving thermal cauterization for pain management.

Swedana: Sweat-inducing therapies used in Ayurveda to eliminate toxins from the body.

Anuvasana Basti: A type of Ayurvedic enema therapy using oil-based solutions.

Niruha Basti: A type of Ayurvedic enema therapy using herbal decoctions.

Raktamokshana: An Ayurvedic blood-letting therapy used for detoxification and treating various skin and blood disorders.

Tarpana: An Ayurvedic eye treatment using ghee to nourish and strengthen the eyes.

Acharya: A spiritual teacher or guide in the Ayurvedic tradition.

Dravya: Substances or materials used in Ayurveda, including herbs, metals, and animal products.

Pitta-vardhaka: Foods, activities or substances that increase the Pitta dosha in the body.

Kapha-vardhaka: Foods, activities or substances that increase the Kapha dosha in the body.

Vata-vardhaka: Foods, activities or substances that increase the Vata dosha in the body.

Srotas: The channels in the body through which the fundamental elements and doshas flow.

Mala: Waste products of the body, such as feces, urine, and sweat.

Sadvritta: Ethical conduct or moral duties in Ayurveda, including personal hygiene and social ethics.

Aushadha: Medicines or drugs in Ayurveda.

Ahar: Diet or food, considered one of the three pillars of life in Ayurveda.

Vihara: Lifestyle practices or routine, considered one of the three pillars of life in Ayurveda.

Nidra: Sleep, considered one of the three pillars of life in Ayurveda.

Vyayama: Physical exercise, an important aspect of a balanced lifestyle in Ayurveda.

Ahara Varga: Classification of foods in Ayurveda based on their properties and effects on the body.

Manas: The mind or mental faculty in Ayurveda, considered the site of cognition and emotion.

Asana: The Sanskrit term for "pose" or "posture". It refers to the physical exercises practiced in yoga.

Pranayama: The practice of controlling the breath in yoga, which is believed to control the energy within the body.

Surya Namaskar: Translates to "Sun Salutation". It's a sequence of 12 yoga poses often used to warm up.

Tadasana: Also known as the "Mountain Pose". It is a basic standing pose used to improve posture, balance, and focus.

Adho Mukha Svanasana: Known as the "Downward-Facing Dog". This pose stretches the whole body and is often used as a transitional pose.

Uttanasana: "Standing Forward Bend". This pose helps to stretch the hamstrings and calm the mind.

Chaturanga Dandasana: Known as the "Four-Limbed Staff Pose". It is a challenging pose that strengthens the arms and abdominal muscles.

Savasana: The "Corpse Pose". Used for relaxation at the end of a yoga practice.

Balasana: Known as the "Child's Pose". It is a resting pose that helps to calm the mind.

Bhujangasana: The "Cobra Pose". This backbend opens the chest and strengthens the spine.

Vrikshasana: Known as the "Tree Pose". A standing balance pose that promotes concentration and balance.

Virabhadrasana: The "Warrior Pose". There are three variations (Warrior I, II, and III), all of which strengthen the legs and arms, improve balance, and open the chest.

Nadi Shodhana: Also known as "Alternate Nostril Breathing". A pranayama technique used to balance the energy in the body.

Kapalabhati: A "Skull Shining Breath". It is a pranayama technique used to cleanse the body and mind.

Ujjayi Pranayama: Known as the "Victorious Breath" or "Ocean Breath". This pranayama technique helps to calm the mind and warm the body.

Mudra: Symbolic or ritual gestures in Hinduism and Buddhism. Often used in meditation or pranayama practice.

Bandha: Internal body locks used in yoga to direct the flow of energy.

Mula Bandha: The "Root Lock". An energetic lock at the base of the spine used in yoga practices.

Uddiyana Bandha: The "Upward Abdominal Lock". This bandha is used in yoga to strengthen the core and promote inner heat.

Jalandhara Bandha: The "Throat Lock". Used in yoga practices to control the flow of energy in the neck area.

Hatha Yoga: A branch of yoga that emphasizes physical exercises to master the body along with mind exercises to withdraw it from external objects.

Vinyasa Yoga: A style of yoga characterized by stringing postures together so that you move from one to another, seamlessly, using breath.

Ashtanga Yoga: A system of yoga recorded by the sage Vamana Rishi in the Yoga Korunta, an ancient manuscript.

Kundalini Yoga: A type of yoga that involves chanting, singing, breathing exercises, and repetitive poses. Its purpose is to activate your Kundalini energy.

Iyengar Yoga: A type of Hatha Yoga that emphasizes detail, precision, and alignment in the performance of postures.

Bikram Yoga: Also known as hot yoga, it's a series of 26 challenging poses performed in a room heated to a high temperature.

Yin Yoga: A slow-paced style of yoga, incorporating principles of traditional Chinese medicine, with postures that are held for longer periods of time.

Restorative Yoga: A practice that is all about slowing down and opening your body through passive stretching.

Patanjali's Eight Limbs of Yoga: The eightfold path of Yoga outlined by Patanjali in the Yoga Sutras. It includes Yama, Niyama, Asana, Pranayama, Pratyahara, Dharana, Dhyana, and Samadhi.

Samadhi: The eighth limb of yoga, defined as a state of ecstasy. The mind becomes still, one-pointed or concentrated while the person remains conscious.

Dhyana: Meditation or total absorption into the object upon that the subject is meditating.

Pratyahara: Withdrawal of the senses, meaning that we make a conscious effort to draw our awareness away from the external world and outside stimuli.

Dharana: Concentration or focusing of the mind.

Yama: Moral codes, which are universal practices.

Niyama: Rules or laws prescribed from observance by the individual.

Bhakti Yoga: A spiritual path or spiritual practice within Hinduism focused on loving devotion towards any personal deity.

Jnana Yoga: The path of knowledge and the practice of mental discipline.

Karma Yoga: The path of selfless service. It teaches to act without being attached to the fruits of one's deeds.

Samskara: Mental and emotional patterns or conditioning that influences our actions and experiences.

Vinyasa: The movement between poses in yoga, typically accompanied by regulated breathing.

Drishti: The focused gaze in a yoga pose, intended to increase mindfulness and balance.

Mantra: A word or phrase repeated to aid concentration in meditation.

Om: A mystic syllable, considered the most sacred mantra in Hinduism and Tibetan Buddhism. It appears at the beginning and end of most Sanskrit recitations, prayers, and texts.

Lotus Pose (Padmasana): An important seated asana in yoga, meditation, and pranayama (breathing exercises).

Bridge Pose (Setu Bandha Sarvangasana): A rejuvenating backbend and common posture in many yoga styles.

Plow Pose (Halasana): A posture that strengthens and opens up the neck, shoulders, abs and back muscles.

Fish Pose (Matsyasana): A pose that stretches and stimulates the muscles of the belly and front of the neck.

Camel Pose (Ustrasana): A backbend that stretches the whole front of the body, particularly the chest, abdomen, quadriceps, and hip flexors.

Cat-Cow Pose (Marjaryasana-Bitilasana): A simple sequence of two poses that warms the body and brings flexibility to the spine.

Eagle Pose (Garudasana): A standing balance pose that requires and develops focus, strength, and serenity.

Diabetes Mellitus: A chronic disease characterized by high blood sugar levels due to the body's inability to produce or effectively use insulin.

Hypertension: Also known as high blood pressure, it's a condition in which the force of blood against the artery walls is too high.

Chronic Arthritis: An umbrella term for conditions causing inflammation and pain in the joints. Includes osteoarthritis, rheumatoid arthritis, gout, etc.

Dementia: A general term for a decline in mental ability severe enough to interfere with daily life. Alzheimer's is the most common type of dementia.

Chronic Asthma: A condition in which a person's airways become inflamed, narrow and swell, and produce extra mucus, making it difficult to breathe.

COPD (Chronic Obstructive Pulmonary Disease): A group of lung diseases that block airflow and make it difficult to breathe.

Migraine: A neurological condition that's characterized by intense, debilitating headaches, often accompanied by nausea, vomiting, and sensitivity to light and sound.

Inflammatory Bowel Disease (IBD): An umbrella term used to describe disorders that involve chronic inflammation of the digestive tract, such as Crohn's disease and ulcerative colitis.

Irritable Bowel Syndrome (IBS): A common disorder that affects the large intestine and causes symptoms like cramping, abdominal pain, bloating, gas, diarrhea, and constipation.

Obesity: A complex disorder involving an excessive amount of body fat. Obesity isn't just a cosmetic concern. It increases the risk of diseases and health problems.

Chronic Eczema: A condition that makes the skin red and itchy. It's common in children but can occur at any age.

Dysmenorrhea: Painful menstrual periods, which can include severe cramps.

Chronic Fatigue Syndrome (CFS): A complicated disorder characterized by extreme fatigue that can't be explained by any underlying medical condition.

SLE (Systemic Lupus Erythematosus): An autoimmune disease in which the body's immune system mistakenly attacks healthy tissue in many parts of the body.

Multiple Sclerosis: A potentially disabling disease of the brain and spinal cord (central nervous system).

Fibromyalgia: A disorder characterized by widespread musculoskeletal pain accompanied by fatigue, sleep, memory, and mood issues.

Hypothyroidism: A condition in which the thyroid gland doesn't produce enough thyroid hormone.

Hyperthyroidism: The overproduction of a hormone by the butterfly-shaped gland in the neck (thyroid).

Anxiety Disorder: A mental health disorder characterized by feelings of worry, anxiety, or fear that are strong enough to interfere with one's daily activities.

Depression: A mood disorder that causes a persistent feeling of sadness and loss of interest.

ADHD (Attention Deficit Hyperactivity Disorder): A chronic condition including attention difficulty, hyperactivity, and impulsiveness.

Insomnia: A sleep disorder that is characterized by difficulty falling and/or staying asleep.

Anorexia Nervosa: An eating disorder characterized by an intense fear of gaining weight and a distorted body image which results in self-imposed starvation and excessive weight loss.

Allergies: Overreaction of the body's immune system to a usually harmless substance.

Alzheimer's Disease: Progressive mental deterioration that can occur in middle or old age, due to generalized degeneration of the brain.

Parkinson's Disease: A progressive nervous system disorder that affects movement.

Sciatica: Pain that radiates along the path of the sciatic nerve, which branches from your lower back through your hips and buttocks and down each leg.

Prostatic Hypertrophy: Also known as BPH (benign prostatic hyperplasia), it's an enlarged prostate gland that can cause urinary symptoms.

Urinary Tract Infections (UTIs): Infections that can happen anywhere along the urinary tract.

Seborrhea: A skin condition that causes a red, itchy, and flaky scalp.

Nephrotic Syndrome: A kidney disorder that causes the body to excrete too much protein in the urine.

Acne: A skin condition that occurs when hair follicles plug with oil and dead skin cells.

Vision Problems: Includes conditions like myopia (nearsightedness), hyperopia (farsightedness), and astigmatism.

Heart Failure: A condition in which the heart can't pump enough blood to meet the body's needs.

Hepatitis: An inflammation of the liver. The condition can be self-limiting or can progress to fibrosis (scarring), cirrhosis, or liver cancer.

Autism: A developmental disorder impairing the ability to communicate and interact.

Osteoporosis: A condition in which bones become weak and brittle.

Drug Addiction: A disease that affects a person's brain and behavior and leads to an inability to control the use of a legal or illegal drug or medication.

Chronic Pain: Persistent or recurrent pain lasting longer than 3-6 months.

Gastroesophageal Reflux Disease (GERD): A chronic digestive disease where stomach acid or, occasionally, stomach content, flows back into the esophagus.

Peptic Ulcer: Open sores that develop on the inside lining of your stomach and the upper portion of your small intestine.

Psoriasis: A common skin condition that speeds up the life cycle of skin cells causing cells to build up rapidly on the surface of the skin.

Menopause: The time that marks the end of your menstrual cycles.

Polycystic Ovary Syndrome (PCOS): A hormonal disorder common among women of reproductive age.

Epilepsy: A central nervous system (neurological) disorder in which brain activity becomes abnormal, causing seizures or periods of unusual behavior, sensations, and sometimes loss of awareness.

Stroke: A medical condition in which poor blood flow to the brain results in cell death.

Atherosclerosis: The build-up of fats, cholesterol, and other substances in and on the artery walls.

Cystic Fibrosis: An inherited disorder that causes severe damage to the lungs, digestive system, and other organs in the body.

Rheumatoid Arthritis: A chronic inflammatory disorder affecting many joints, including those in the hands and feet.

Chronic Kidney Disease (CKD): Long-term loss of kidney function which can lead to end-stage kidney disease or kidney failure.

Printed in Great Britain
by Amazon

24582507R00136